CLINICAL COMMUNICATION HANDBOOK

CLINICAL COMMUNICATION HANDBOOK

Melissa Piasecki, MD
Associate Professor
Department of Psychiatry and Behavioral Science
University of Nevada School of Medicine
Reno, Nevada

Blackwell
Publishing

Blackwell Publishing, Inc., 350 Main Street, Malden, Massachusetts 02148-5018, USA
Blackwell Science Ltd., Osney Mead, Oxford OX2 0EL, UK
Blackwell Science Asia Pty Ltd, 550 Swanston Street, Carlton, Victoria 3053, Australia
Blackwell Verlag GmbH, Kurfürstendamm 57, 10707 Berlin, Germany

02 03 04 05 5 4 3 2 1

ISBN: 0-632-04646-5

Library of Congress Cataloging-in-Publication Data

Piasecki, Melissa.
Clinical communication handbook / by Melissa Piasecki.
p. ; cm.
Includes bibliographical references.
ISBN 0-632-04646-5 (pbk.)
1. Communication in medicine. 2. Medical personnel and patient. 3. Physician and patient.
[DNLM: 1. Communication. 2. Physician-Patient Relations. W 62 P581c 2002] I. Title.
R118 .P535 2002
610.69'6—dc21

2002003791

A catalogue record for this title is available from the British Library

Acquisitions: Beverly Copland
Development: Julia Casson
Production: Debra Lally
Cover design: Hannus Design
Typesetter: Graphicraft Limited in Hong Kong
Printed and bound by Sheridan Books in Chelsea, MI, USA

For further information on Blackwell Publishing, visit our website:
www.blackwellscience.com

Table of Contents

Preface

This text is a handbook for all students and clinicians. Although the word "physician" is regularly used, a number of other clinical roles could easily substitute. For example, nursing, physician assistant, or pharmacy students and professionals are an important part of the intended readership. Excellent communication skills complement anyone's clinical interactions. In addition, this is a useful text for students preparing for their clinical skills assessments with patients.

In *Clinical Communication Handbook,* I aim to present the "A to Z"s of communication. This includes basics on professionalism (such as dress) as well as the challenges of empathy and compassion. Some of these topics will be self-evident to certain readers and lifelong challenges to others. I personally have found students in medicine to vary widely in the type of feedback and support that is most helpful to them. This book attempts to be as useful as possible by presenting a wide range of information, knowing that self-learners will pick and choose what they need. The vignettes and dialogue in this text are generally composites of different patient encounters and are not specific to any one person.

The Bayer Institute in Health Care Communications developed part of the content of this text in the "Clinician–Patient Communication" workshop manual. The Institute's "E4" and "coaching" models have been widely disseminated in training workshops. I have made every attempt to accurately reference this material to the 1998 workshop manual. Keller and Carroll are to be credited with introducing the "E4" model in their 1994 publication "A new model for physician-patient communication." One of the goals for writing this book was to make this material available to students and others who may not ordinarily have the opportunity to participate in the workshops. Another goal was to adopt the Bayer Institute's philosophy of using evidence-based approaches to teaching communication skills and to expand the scope of the workshop material.

Melissa Piasecki
April 2002

Acknowledgments

Some ideas for this book borrow generously from conversations with my academic colleagues Barbara Kohlenberg, David Antonuccio, and Elizabeth Gifford. I wish to thank the physicians and nurses who provided me and my family with an understanding of the power and value of empathy and compassion. I also wish to thank the editorial staff at Blackwell Publishing for their assistance and support in developing this text. A special thank you to Elizabeth Athens for her assistance in this and other projects. Thanks to Joe Phelan for all of his love and support.

Reviewers

Keith Chan
Class of 2003
Stanford University
Stanford, California

Brandon Johnson
Internal Medicine resident
Baptist Hospital
Birmingham, Alabama

Nancy Panhdi
Family Practice resident
Shenandoah Family Practice Residency
Front Royal, Virginia

Derek Wayman
Class of 2003
University of North Dakota
Grand Forks, North Dakota

For Joseph, Elizabeth Rose and Leo

1

Communication Is Critical

Today's medical student learns a long list of procedures to become a physician—auscultation and percussion, the rectal exam, and lumbar puncture to name a few. All of these involve important skills which are taught and learned so that doctors can provide competent medical care. However, the single procedure that is most often used and is the most critical to patient care is rarely described as a procedure—the patient interview. The necessary skills for this procedure are communication skills. A typical career in clinical medicine includes over 100,000 patient interviews (1). Communication—both verbal and nonverbal—is central to every clinical encounter and may be one of the most important factors in patient care and medical outcomes.

As with the examination procedures mentioned above, communication is a *skill.* The techniques can be learned as a student and mastered over time. Most students do not get the same type of clear, systematic guidance in learning communication skills as they do with other procedures. As a result, many experience less confidence and more anxiety when talking to patients than when they draw blood or examine reflexes. Difficult situations and certain patients present bigger challenges for most students and clinicians. Fortunately, specific, learnable skills are available for all types of physician–patient interactions.

It is important that students and doctors feel comfortable and competent in their work, and effective communication skills can make this possible. There are a number of additional benefits to having such skills, and the following sections describe some of the research findings on how these skills can improve specific medical outcomes for patients and positively affect malpractice rates, patient satisfaction, and doctor job satisfaction (1).

MEDICAL OUTCOMES

Most physicians are highly motivated to help patients get better. As a goal-oriented group, physicians tend to place more emphasis on treatment effectiveness than on other factors listed in later sections of this chapter. A surprisingly wide variety of medical outcomes improve as a result of effective physician communication. Different communication techniques such as positive suggestion, enhanced education, and emotional care (physicians offering warmth, appropriate reassurance, and empathy) have all been shown to have a positive impact on patients' health status. Physicians "who attempted to form warm, friendly relationships with their patients, who reassured them . . . were found to be more effective than practitioners who kept their consultations impersonal, formal, or uncertain" (2). Examples of improved medical outcomes include improvements in headaches, postsurgical pain, blood pressure, and glucose control (3). Improved medical outcomes in some patients may be related to their adherence (also known as compliance) with prescribed treatment—the better the relationship with the physician, the more likely the patient will feel confident about the treatment plan and take medications as prescribed. The topic of patient adherence to treatment regimens is discussed in greater detail in Chapter 7 on "enlisting" the patient.

PATIENT SATISFACTION

> Communication is the most important variable in the physician–patient relationship. It drives consumer perception

that high quality medical care is being received as well as overall satisfaction with physician relationships. (4)

Although the majority of patients and physicians are generally satisfied with their relationships, the number one complaint patients have about physicians is "poor communication." Not surprisingly, overall patient satisfaction is highest when a physician is a skilled communicator (4). Patient satisfaction does not reflect only the physician's communication behavior. Research shows that some characteristics of patients (such as individual preferences and attitudes about health care) and of the health care setting (parking, waiting room, and reception and nursing staff) also impact the patients' reports of satisfaction.

Physician communication does play a large role, however. Specific physician behaviors such as "partnership building" (see Chapters 6 and 7) and "social emotional behavior" (see Chapters 4 and 5) were positively related to patient satisfaction in a review of 41 studies (5).

PHYSICIAN SATISFACTION

Medical school and residency training programs are intensive and expensive life investments for the people who complete them. Most trainees accept the costs and burdens of their training because they expect a very high level of satisfaction in their careers as physicians. Higher ratings of job satisfaction among physicians appear to be closely linked to good relationships—and therefore to good communication skills—with patients.

Physician satisfaction has been evaluated from the perspective of both individual office visits with patients and global career satisfaction. In either case, physicians rated the relationships they had with patients as important factors in feeling good about their careers. Positive and friendly exchanges and the use of humor with patients led physicians to rate individual patient encounters as more satisfying (6).

When asked to report on global satisfaction with their careers, doctors from a variety of specialties rated "good relationships with patients, relatives, and staff" as the greatest contributors to job satisfaction. These positive relationships are particularly important as adequate job satisfaction appears to protect physicians from the negative effects of job stress. "Burnout" and psychiatric problems in physicians are less common when job satisfaction is high (7). In addition, physicians who describe themselves as inadequately trained in communication skills have a higher rate of burnout (8). A 1995 survey confirmed that physicians who feel good about their patient communication skills are twice as likely to be very satisfied with their overall patient relationships (compared to physicians who are not satisfied with their skills) (4).

MALPRACTICE

All physicians make mistakes. Not all physicians get sued. Research has examined the differences between the clinicians who are named in malpractice suits and those who are not. The most important factor that determines why patients sue their physicians is relationship (i.e., communication) problems.

In a sample of 45 plaintiff depositions, researchers identified "relationship issues" that appeared to be central to 71% of the lawsuits. Some examples of the problems described in the depositions were how a clinician returned phone calls, listened to patient problems, gave information, or managed a family's grief. The plaintiffs described the physicians they were suing as arrogant, devaluing, unavailable, or abandoning (9).

Another study of malpractice examined whether the obstetricians who had a greater than average number of malpractice claims against them had provided a lower quality of technical care to their patients. The researchers reviewed the medical records 5 or 10 years later from a group of physicians with a higher than average number

BOX 1.1
Communication Skills

Benefits to Patient

Better results from medical treatment
Greater satisfaction with medical care

Benefits to Physician

Greater job satisfaction and less "burnout"
Better relationships with patients
Lower malpractice risk

of malpractice claims, as compared with a control group of obstetricians with no malpractice claims or an average number of claims. They found no difference in the number of technical or clinical errors among these groups, suggesting that some other factor other than bad outcome was driving some patients to sue their obstetricians (10). Looking for other factors, the same investigators interviewed women patients of obstetricians who had a history of greater than average malpractice claims and compared their responses with patients of a control group of obstetricians. They found that the sued obstetricians were not more likely to have bad pregnancy outcomes, but they did have significantly greater numbers of patient complaints and decreased patient satisfaction compared to the control group obstetricians. Women were more likely to be dissatisfied about poor patient–physician communication; they described feelings of being rushed during appointments, and of their doctor not listening to them, and, at times, of being "yelled at." The obstetricians who had never been sued were described by patients as more caring and more willing to communicate (11).

Looking at other physician groups, researchers have found that primary care physicians with a history of no malpractice claims had significant differences in communication style compared to physicians who had a history of claims. The "no claims" physicians spent on average 3.3

minutes more with patients and engaged and enlisted with them more (12).

Although avoiding malpractice claims is not the main reason why most students or doctors should seek to develop and master communication skills, research strongly suggests that good skills decrease malpractice risk by improving relationships and patient satisfaction.

KEY POINTS

1. More than any other specific skill, technique, or procedure in patient care, good communication skills are critical in helping patients get better.
2. More satisfaction for patients and physicians, lower "burnout" rates among physicians, and decreased malpractice risk are added benefits to good communication skills.
3. Students, residents, and physicians often lack teaching, training, and practice in this critical area.

This book offers some practical ideas and a systematic approach to any patient encounter (time management, the four "E's," closing) (13). Additional discussion is devoted to getting feedback on skills and on situations that may require special communication strategies. With a clear approach to communication and the opportunity to practice their skills, all clinicians can develop their potential as highly effective and satisfied physicians.

REFERENCES

1. Bayer Institute for Health Care Communication. Clinician–patient communication to enhance health outcomes: a workshop manual. West Haven, CT: Bayer Institute, 1998.
2. Di Blasi Z, Harkness E, Ernst E, et al. Influence of context on health outcomes: a systematic review. Lancet 2001;357:757–762.
3. Stewart MS. Effective physician–patient communication and health outcomes: a review. Can Med Assoc J 1995;152:1423–1433.

4. Worthlin Group. Communication and the physician/patient relationship: a physician and consumer communication survey. West Haven, CT: Bayer Institute for Health Care Communication, 1995.
5. Hall JA, Roter DL, Katz NR. Meta-analysis of correlates of provider behavior in medical encounters. Med Care 1988;26: 657–675.
6. Suchman AL, Roter D, Green M, et al. Physician satisfaction with primary care office visits. Med Care 1993;31:1083–1092.
7. Ramirez AJ, Graham J, Richards MA, et al. Mental health of hospital consultants: the effects of stress and satisfaction at work. Lancet 1996;347:724–728.
8. Graham J, Ramirez AJ. Mental health of hospital consultants. J Psychosom Res 1997;43:227–231.
9. Beckman HB, Markakis KM, Suchman AL, Frankel RM. The doctor–patient relationship and malpractice: lessons from plaintiff depositions. Arch Intern Med 1994;154:1365–1370.
10. Entman SS, Glass CA, Hickson GB, et al. The relationship between malpractice claims history and subsequent obstetric care. JAMA 1994;272:1588–1591.
11. Hickson GB, Clyton EW, Entman SS, et al. Obstetricians' prior malpractice experience and patients' satisfaction with care. JAMA 1994;272:1583–1588.
12. Levinson W, Roter DL, Mullooly JP, et al. Physician–patient communication: the relationship with malpractice claims among primary care physicians and surgeons. JAMA 1997;277:553–559.
13. Keller VF, Carroll JG. A new model for physician–patient communication. Patient Educ Couns 1994;23:134–140.

2

Getting Started

This chapter is about the basics—how to most effectively enter into the role of physician. Despite old stereotypes of the middle-aged white male physician in a white coat and tie, medical professionals today are multicultural and of all shapes, sizes, and styles. No one should give up his or her individual flair to fit into a preconceived image role of the "medical professional." In fact, it is the most real and human elements about a physician that allow for meaningful relationships to build with patients. This chapter will address the image (both appearance and behavior) of the physician and how students and doctors can (and should) preserve their individuality while maintaining professionalism and interpersonal effectiveness.

Studies of physician effectiveness, which measure outcomes such as patient satisfaction and the need for emergency medical treatments, demonstrate that there are no demographic (age, gender, race, etc.) advantages in medicine. This means that, as a group, older black women doctors are no more or less effective than young Asian male doctors or middle-aged Hispanic women doctors. The gender, age, and ethnicity of physicians do not effect their potential ability to provide excellent and effective care. An individual's physical appearance and behavior, however, can sometimes have a dramatic impact on the patient–physician relationship.

APPEARANCE

First impressions typically form in a few seconds and endure a long time. For a physician, appearance and mannerisms are the basis on which patients form their first impressions. There is a wide spectrum of clothing and personal grooming styles that are appropriate for the hospital and clinic. Dress and styles that fall outside of this spectrum are likely to distract the patient and detract from the physician's effectiveness. Some hospitals and medical schools have "dress codes" or guidelines, but many do not. Below are some suggestions for staying within the professional spectrum.

Always wear an identification badge when interacting with patients. This is probably the most important tool any professional has for establishing his or her role. Photo IDs are best. The name on the badge should be printed large enough for someone to read when sitting a few feet away. The badge should also include title or position (e.g., "Medical Student," "Resident in Surgery," or "Psychiatrist"). Many patients in the hospital or a busy clinic cannot catch the names or roles of their physicians during the initial introduction and will check the name badge a few times to make sure they know to whom they are talking. The white coat is also an important tool in communicating one's role. Patients perceive clinicians in white coats as more "hygienic, professional, authoritative, scientific, competent, knowledgeable, and approachable" (1).

Commit to maintaining a standard of appearance. This implies a freshly washed/shaven, professionally dressed appearance each morning. Physicians and medical students work the longest hours and have some of the most demanding and erratic schedules of any career. Ironically, they are also the professionals most in need of presenting a consistent, professional appearance. Sometimes a shave and shower will cut into precious sleep time and an ironed shirt may seem an impossibility. However, basic standards of appearance have a dramatic impact on patients' impressions, and the time invested to maintain the standard is paid off in effectiveness with patients. The unshaven intern with "bed head" and an untucked shirt is unlikely to inspire much confidence in patients or their families. The third-year resident with "big" hair and evidence of her last meal and blood draw on her white coat may not be able to get the attention of her patient.

There is a wide range of clothing seen among physicians in hospitals and clinics. The "casual Friday" culture has led to a wonderful acceptance and availability of khakis and sporty shirts to match. Unless there is an institutional dress code that specifies otherwise, khakis and short-sleeved shirts are appropriate for patient care, as long as they are clean, not wrinkled, and accompanied by a white coat with a name badge. Khakis represent the minimum in professional dress. More formal dress (slacks, skirts, dress shirts) may be more fitting in certain environments. Observations of the "culture" in an institution—that is, how the more senior professionals dress—is a good way to plan wardrobe. Denim and tee-shirts, even on weekends, communicate an unprofessional image. Scrubs are a better alternative and can be worn with athletic shoes.

There are some problems in dress that are specific to women (see Vignette 2.1). Short skirts and midriff exposure are mainstream styles that do not work well in the clinical setting. Even longer skirts sometimes have slits that expose the midthigh. Certain patient populations—such as adolescents, some psychiatric patients, and elderly patients—will be distracted and may misinterpret revealing clothing. In general, more coverage of the chest and upper legs is better. A doctor's surgical scrubs can fall open when she leans over, exposing the entire chest. Women need to check out the fit of a scrub top ahead of time and may need to wear a close-fitting shirt underneath. Sheer fabrics or clingy knits sometimes do not provide adequate coverage of breasts. A blazer or sweater may be necessary to maintain a professional appearance if a white coat is not worn. Some women medical students find that they are less likely to be identified in the physician's role than are their male colleagues. To reduce the risk of non-identification as a physician or medical student, women

CLINICAL VIGNETTE 2.1

MD: Sue, I'd like a few moments of your time now that we're finished with rounds.
Student: Sure. Did I do something wrong?
MD: No—your workups and patient presentations are great. There was something else I wanted to mention to you. You are a very good student but I think your style of dressing could be a distraction to the patients.
Student: What do you mean?
MD: I've noticed two things in the last week. You wore a skirt the other day—I think it was red—that revealed more of your leg than you probably were aware of. Your patient with pancreatitis never made eye contact with you on rounds—he was staring at your skirt. And today I think your blouse is pretty sheer and exposes more than is appropriate for patient care.
Student: Wow. I feel really awful.
MD: This isn't about making you feel bad, it's about alerting you about what may or may not be professional dress. I always wear either a blazer or white coat to avoid the problems with blouses—it also makes me feel more like a physician. And I gave up on skirts long ago after my first code in the hospital—skirts and CPR don't mix too well. Can I suggest a catalog that has comfortable women's clothes that seem to work well for hospital and clinic work?

can wear a white coat and name badge and avoid white or pastel clothing (which may more typically be worn by allied health professionals).

One particular problem that can arise for individuals at any level and from any background is body odor (see Vignette 2.2). Typically, a daily shower with deodorant soap followed by an antiperspirant and a clean shirt completely manages this problem, which could otherwise undermine

CLINICAL VIGNETTE 2.2

MD 1: Jeremy, can I ask you something personal?
MD 2: Sure, what's up?
MD 1: Well, I have a question in my mind about how I appear to my patients and colleagues, and I was wondering if I could ask you about it.
MD 2: What sort of question?
MD 1: Do you think that I could ever be offensive in my appearance or body odor?
MD 2: Whoa—that *is* personal!
MD 1: Yes, but I'm not certain about it, and I really need to ask someone who can tell me honestly.
MD 2: Honestly, Bill, there are mornings when you are looking pretty scruffy. And sometimes on weekends the nurses comment that you seem to have had a "great workout" that morning. It seems that there may be times when you need to hit the showers before doing patient rounds. One thing I noticed—there's never any soap in the on-call showers. But you can always grab a bar from the patient supply closet on 2C.
MD 1: That's really helpful. I appreciate you talking to me about this.

relationships with patients (and colleagues). If there is any question in one's mind about body odor, he or she may consider asking frank and supportive colleagues if they have ever noticed a problem or heard of others noticing any problems. Strong-smelling perfume or cologne can offend as well, and can even trigger nausea in pregnant or chemotherapy patients.

Related to the problem of body odor is breath odor. During parts of a physical exam, such as the eye exam, the physician is face to face with patients. Clinical interviews usually occur at an interpersonal distance that is close enough to transmit bad breath odors. Most clinicians have had the uncomfortable experience sitting in the chair of a dentist or hair stylist who has bad breath. Some breath odor is related to certain foods—garlic in the Caesar salad from lunch, for example. At other times, it is related to dental problems or genetics. As with body odor, the key factor is recognition, which usually only occurs when a direct question is asked of a supportive colleague, such as "I have been eating at the new Italian restaurant—do you think I have garlic breath?" Sometimes well-intentioned friends and colleagues will offer breath mints or mint gum without ever directly bringing up the topic. An offer of a breath mint might be an important hint that needs to be directly addressed. Regardless of how a physician learns of a breath problem, he or she will need to start a mouth hygiene routine at home and at the office that includes brushing teeth after all meals, and using a mouthwash after brushing. If the problems persist, then breath spray (used in between clinical encounters) and a dental exam may help. Gum and mints used during patient care are distracting and relay an unprofessional image.

MAINTAINING INDIVIDUALITY

No one wants to be stripped of his or her individuality—the things that make us special or different. An important skill in medicine is to preserve one's uniqueness in a way that does not distract from the role of physician. Examples of ways to maintain a sense of self-identity include keeping a designer (or amusing) pen in the pocket, wearing buttons on the white coat, and/or adding personal touches to the clipboard such as stickers, calendars, or family photos. Men can wear colorful ties (with cartoons, if working around children), keep a small earring in a previously pierced ear, wear festive socks, and wear long hair tied back. Women can add pins to the lapel of the white coat, or wear colorful scrubs, bright scarves, or interesting jewelry (see Vignette 2.3). In general, tattoos and body jewelry (nose, brow, or lip rings) are distracting to patients and

CLINICAL VIGNETTE 2.3

Patient: Excuse me, Doctor, but what is that pin you are wearing?
MD: Oh, that's "The Owl and the Pussycat" from a children's poem. Did you ever hear of it?
Patient: Yes, it was a favorite of my kids.
MD: My child too. So I wear it for fun when I see pediatric patients.

are best minimized or concealed. For physician smokers, their cigarette use can send patients mixed messages; concealing all evidence of tobacco use (including smoke on the breath) will project the best possible image to patients.

What makes us individuals also makes us interesting. Patients will naturally be curious and want to ask questions about what we reveal about ourselves. In a later section there are examples of how to manage personal inquiries from patients.

BEHAVIOR

Just as first impressions are made with appearances, so the same is true of physician behaviors. The goal for professionalism is the same—to maintain a professional role while allowing individuality. Later chapters describe in detail a number of specific behaviors to welcome and engage a patient. In this chapter, the emphasis is on general physician behaviors, with an emphasis on nonverbal communication.

Make eye contact and smile. Within the first two seconds of being in a room with a patient, the physician needs to seek eye contact and smile. Lapses on the physician's part communicate disinterest (and possibly disrespect) to the patient.

CLINICAL VIGNETTE 2.4

Patient: Doctor, how do you say your name?
MD: Piasecki. It's actually spelled almost phonetically. Here, I'll give you one of the clinic cards and I'll circle it.
Patient: Thanks.

Introduce self and role. Even if it is evident who the physician is and what he or she is doing, most patients appreciate hearing it repeated for the first few encounters (see Vignette 2.4). Medical students in particular need to orient the patient to their role. An example is "Hi. I'm Jamie. I'm a medical student at the university here and I'm here to interview you about your medical history." Simple introductions usually work best—terms such as "second-year preceptor student," "clinical research fellow," or "con-sulting attending psychiatrist" can confuse most patients. Using the term "student" or "doctor" orients most patients, as in combinations such as "medical student in surgery" or "psychiatry doctor." A visible name badge reinforces the introduction and can give the patient a chance to see how the name is spelled. Many patients will ask a physician to spell his or her name; writing it out on a piece of paper (or even on a box of tissue at the bedside) will only take a few seconds and is usually greatly appreciated.

Speak clearly. A physician's time is his or her most precious commodity. Time pressure can tempt someone to speak a little faster or less clearly—and make it easy to miss the perplexed expression on a patient's face. Regional and national accents can also make it more difficult for patients to understand what their physician is saying (see Vignette 2.5). Some patients—those who are hearing impaired or who are exceptionally anxious—will have a more difficult time following along. Most patients, aware of how busy the physician is, will not ask for information to be repeated, even if they did not understand what was

CLINICAL VIGNETTE 2.5

MD: As I am sure you have noticed, I speak with an Indian accent that can make it hard for my patients to understand what I say. Please let me know as we go along if you do not understand something I say and I will explain it better.
Patient: Well, what did you mean by "lavage"?
MD: Oh, that is a medical term that means to wash or flush. It's usually when we have to rinse out a patient's stomach. "Pumping the stomach" is another expression we use.
Patient: And what did you mean when you said something about "I see you"?
MD: The Intensive Care Unit—or ICU. That is where you may be admitted after the emergency room for more medical care.

said. If a physician is aware that he or she has an accent, it is helpful to acknowledge that early on in the encounter and invite the patient to ask for clarifications.

Background noise or music and bright backlighting also can make it difficult for patients to follow a physician's speech. Whenever possible, the physician should turn off the television or radio in a hospital room, close the door or curtains, and take a position that enables the patient to optimally see as well as hear everything that is said.

Wash hands. If a room in an office or a hospital room has a sink, the physician needs to wash his or her hands before touching the patient (including shaking the patient's hand). Some medical schools will automatically fail a student on a clinical exam if the student forgets this. After practicing hand washing "first thing" for a few months, it will become a habit for a physician and eventually automatic. Ideally, the sink should not be positioned so that the physician must turn his or her back on the patient.

CLINICAL VIGNETTE 2.6

MD: Hello, Mrs. Baker—how are you today?
Patient: Oh, call me "Angeline."
MD: Great. Angeline, what can I do for you today?

Strategically located sinks allow physicians to make eye contact and verbally interact while they are washing their hands. Some medical professionals are very aware of how commonly diseases spread in hospitals and will remind their own physicians to wash their hands if they do not see them do it upon entering the exam room.

Shake hands. A friendly, warm, gentle handshake is almost always an appropriate gesture for both new and returning patients. Exceptions are when the patient has an IV line or an injury on that hand, and when the physician has not been able to wash hands since the last patient encounter.

Be formal. Just as a handshake suggests a cordial yet formal relationship, using formal address with a patient is a sign of professionalism and respect. Adult patients generally prefer to be addressed as Mr., Mrs., Ms., or Dr., depending on their life role. Although a patient will rarely complain directly, most find it presumptuous for someone they do not know well to assume a first-name basis. Informal terms, such as "honey" or "sweetie," are potentially degrading as well and suggest a problem with the physician's professional boundaries. Erring on the side of formality is preferable to insulting a patient. Patients who want to be called by their first names will almost always volunteer that information in a friendly way (2) (see Vignette 2.6).

Use gestures. Specific hand and facial gestures can convey a wealth of interpersonal information to a patient. Hands in front, with palms up or fingertips touching, can communicate an active interest in listening to what the patient says. Leaning forward toward the patient, eyebrows slightly raised, also conveys attention and concern. Physicians can send a patient a message that the topic at hand needs special attention by placing hands down on a surface in front of them or pointing toward the patient with both index fingers touching. A universal gesture of warmth or reassurance is a hand on the shoulder or a lingering pat on the back. This nonverbal act communicates support and caring, especially at a time of bad news (3).

Be organized. There is a minimum of necessary organization every physician needs to have when starting a clinical encounter. Fumbling for a pen and running out of the office in search of a billing slip communicate problems with professionalism (and possibly with competency as well). No physician can function without a pen, and placing a few capped pens in the pocket at the beginning of the day can be part of a morning routine. Clipboards and charts (or PDAs) need to be within arm's reach, as do prescription pads and billing slips. Reference materials (formularies, referral sources) should also be at hand.

Be on time. Another aspect of organization that contributes to a patient's first impression is timeliness. A scheduled appointment time can be considered a commitment between a physician and his or her patients. Some practice environments do not allow physicians complete autonomy over scheduling. Whenever possible, a physician's commitment to keeping appointment times will enhance his or her professional image (and decrease the stress of "overcommitment").

WORKING WITH DIFFERENCES

Every medical professional will have some distinguishing feature that will attract attention from patients. It might be an engagement ring, a skin color, or an interesting last name. Patients will always be interested in their physicians and will often express their curiosity with questions. Some inquiries will not appear so benign—they may imply a suspicion of incompetence or express hostility. Often, it is appropriate to respond to the patient's questions with a simple answer, not volunteering any additional personal information. At other times, it may be important to find out what concerns led to the question and provide appropriate responses or reassurances. At other times, it is most appropriate to establish a professional boundary and clarify to the patient that some personal information is not appropriate or comfortable to disclose. In general, minimal disclosure of personal information is most appropriate.

The following scenarios are composites of medical student and physician experiences involving patient inquiries and physician responses. The last section of this chapter offers an opportunity for the reader to form his or her own responses to some common patient inquiries.

1. **Patient:** What kind of name is "Piasecki"?
   Physician: A lot of people ask me that. It's an Eastern European name from my family. Now, I'd like to ask you about your medicines.
   (There is no additional self-disclosure—just a straightforward and limited response to the question, given in a friendly manner, and a redirection of the interview to the patient's history.)

2. **Patient:** (to East Indian physician) Where are you from?
   Physician: I am from India. Sometimes people wonder about my training. Do you have any questions?
   Patient: No, I was curious about where you were from. I know you're a good doctor.
   Physician: Thank you for that compliment!
   (The physician acknowledges his patient's interest and nondefensively invites him to express other questions he may have that reflect a need for more information or reassurance.)

3. **Patient:** (to young female physician) How old are you anyway?
   Physician: That's an interesting question. Why do you ask?

Patient: Well, you seem so young, I can't hardly believe you graduated from college.
Physician: Well, I'm old enough to have been a doctor for six years now, that's for sure. I'd like move on to you, and take a look at your blood pressure record.
Patient: OK.
(The physician does not directly answer this question, although some might. She is able to reassure her patient that she is an experienced and qualified physician. Some youthful looking physicians make a joke about their "pact with the devil." Although this is commonly used, it may not always be appropriate.)

Practice Examples

The reader is invited to respond to the following potential patient inquiries. Some possible responses will follow.

1. **Patient:** (to a female medical student) "Is that an engagement ring?"
   Medical Student: ______________________________
   ____
   ____
   ____
   ____
2. **Patient:** (to a male physician) "You're Jewish, aren't you?"
   Physician: ______________________________
   ____
   ____
   ____
   ____
3. **Patient:** (to a female physician) "Are you pregnant?!"
   Physician: ______________________________
   ____
   ____
   ____
   ____

Sample Responses

1. "Yes, it is an engagement ring. I'm getting married in May. Thank you for noticing. Now, let's get back to your concerns for this visit." (Denying or deflecting a question about an obvious engagement ring would not make much sense. If you do not want a patient to ask about or comment on obvious jewelry, it would be best to leave the jewelry at home.)

2.
   A. "Well, I tend to not discuss personal things at work, partly because I think the time here is for taking care of patients. I *would* like to find out more about your pain and what we can do for it today."
   B. "Is it important for you to know that?
   C. "My family was Jewish. I don't think of myself as a practicing Jew."
   (If a patient makes a compelling request, some physicians disclose religion, marital status, and other personal information. Some physicians have tight boundaries and consider personal information out of place with patient care. It is usually a balance that factors in the personal style of the physician and the quality of the physician–patient relationship.)

3. "Yes, I am expecting in March. Let's talk at the end of our visit about the time I will be away and who will be covering for me."
   (Questions about pregnancy often have an unvoiced concern attached: "Who will take care of my medical needs while you are out having a baby?" Assuming this unvoiced concern, physicians can reassure patients as soon as the issue arises.)

KEY POINTS

1. A professional appearance involves clothing choices, attention to grooming, and awareness of possible problem areas.

2. Professional behaviors include washing hands, making eye contact, shaking hands, making introductions, and using appropriate formality.
3. Maintaining individuality is entirely consistent with professionalism.
4. Patients will always be curious about their doctors and will ask personal questions. There are a number of effective ways of managing these inquiries.

REFERENCES

1. Gooden BR, Smith MJ, Tattersall SJ, Stockler MR. Hospitalised patients' views on doctors and white coats. Med J Aust 2001;175:219–222.
2. Keller V, Baker L. Communicate with care. RN 2000;63:32–33.
3. Bell AH. More than words can say: what your non-verbal signals say to patients. OU Physician's Res 2000;Nov/Dec:32–37.

3

About Time

The greatest gift a patient can receive from a doctor is the gift of time—specifically the first two minutes of the interview. An investment of two minutes yields tremendous benefits for the interviewer as well, in the quality and quantity of data and in establishing rapport. The beginning minutes of each interview can be the most critical and useful.

Many students and doctors have great difficulty giving patients two or three minutes to fully complete their initial statements. Doctors feel so pressured by time limits that they almost always interrupt their patients very early on in the interview. How early? Resident physicians in one study interrupted their patients after an average of 18 seconds. Of the 52 patients who were interrupted, only one was allowed to later complete his or her sentence (1). A second study with more experienced doctors found that patients were interrupted after 23 seconds (2). Such early interruptions hurt the interview in several ways.

First, patients perceive that their doctors care about them less when they interrupt them early on. It is difficult for the patient to feel that the doctor is truly interested in the patient's concerns when the doctor interrupts the patient's first sentence. (Allowing the patient to tell his or her story will be discussed more in Chapter 5.) A second problem is that early interruptions prevent patients from describing some of the concerns they want to cover during this interview or office visit. Unexpressed concerns can lead to undiagnosed problems. This in turn sets the stage for patient dissatisfaction, inefficient interviews, and poorer medical outcomes. For example, a study of 20 general practitioners examined different types of misunderstandings that could occur in patient–doctor communications. It found that "all misunderstandings were associated with the lack of patients' participation in the consultation." In addition, a review of the misunderstandings revealed that they were medically relevant and associated with worse or potentially worse outcomes for the patients (3).

A third advantage to an uninterrupted, open-ended query at the beginning of the interview is that it can avoid the "doorknob complaint." This is the patient complaint that emerges as the physician places his or her hand on the doorknob to leave the room at the end of the interview: "By the way doctor, I've been feeling weak and dizzy in the morning." Doorknob complaints force the interviewer to either extend the time of the interview, reschedule the patient soon to evaluate this new complaint, or make a hasty assessment and plan of the new problem at hand. Most physicians are uncomfortable with waiting or not fully examining the new problem by extending the office visit —thus, investing two full minutes in the first part of the interview can save time at the very end.

Opening the interview by inviting patients to describe the problems in their own words for the first two minutes effectively lays the groundwork for the type of patient participation that can improve outcomes. It is impossible, however, for many physicians and students to resist the strong urge to interrupt during those first two minutes. At the end of this chapter are some strategies to overcome this urge. Once listening at the beginning becomes part of a physician's routine approach to medical interviewing, the benefits of not interrupting on patient rapport and information gathering should reinforce the technique. Chapter 4, on engaging the patient, shows some examples of open-ended questions that work for beginning an interview.

BOX 3.1

Let's go back to the cough you described—what was coming up while you coughed?
I need to understand more about how you are taking the blood pressure medication—how many pills a day?
As I glance at your chart I see that last time you were here we discussed decreasing the pain medication to two pills a day—how did that work for pain control?
Let me interrupt a minute—I understand that you have been feeling pretty sick for a week. Help me understand why you decided to come into treatment *today?*
I'm afraid I'm a little confused—how does the picnic last weekend fit into today's office visit?

After the first two minutes, the physician is likely to have many questions to expand and clarify what the patient has said. Patients can be redirected by means of open-ended or closed-ended questions. Box 3.1 has a few examples of clarifying questions.

In studies of medical practices in North America, roughly half of patient complaints and problems were missed by their doctors (4). For patients, frequent interruptions may result in reduced satisfaction, less adherence to the prescribed medical regimen, and poorer medical outcomes. Of course, this is not because doctors are incompetent or do not care about patients; rather, it is because doctors have learned to communicate with patients in ways that block the flow of information from the patient to the doctor. Interviewers might be experiencing perceived time pressure; have learned high control interview styles from residents, attending physicians, and other role models during training; or have little specific training on listening skills. A review of 21 articles on doctor–patient communication found that open types of communication improved outcomes in blood pressure, blood sugar, emotional status, pain, and functional status (5). The time-efficient doctor is looking for a chief complaint, but patients only know how to talk about their problems in their own words, in their own way.

GUIDES TO TIME MANAGEMENT

Just as students learn with practice which questions to ask and how to ask them, they must learn how to manage *time* during an interview. This is the interviewer's responsibility—no patient can be expected to keep an eye on the clock for the physician. Here are a few practical recommendations for time management during patient encounters:

1. Give the first two minutes over to the patient. Learn to do this by writing down the time after the first question is asked, then refraining from interrupting the patient until two minutes have passed. (First question: "Mrs. Alberts, what can I do for you today?" Margin note on paper: "Start time 2:15.") Some physicians have trained themselves to wait a full two minutes by using a two-minute egg timer.
2. Before walking into the examining room be clear about what the schedule is like and how much time is allotted to spend with this patient.
3. Have clocks and timepieces visible from the examiner's interview position in the room. A wall clock above the patient's chair or table will allow discreet time checks. Ideally, the clock should be in the same field of vision as the patient's head. Obvious glances at a wristwatch can send a message that the physician is impatient for a visit to be over.
4. Avoid interruptions (phones, pagers) and apologize for any interruptions. ("I am so sorry—I had to take that call and it interrupted our appointment. Let's get back to what you were telling me about the pain on the left side.")

5. Give a five-minute warning when you are concerned about "cutting off" a patient. ("We will have to wrap up today's visit in about five minutes.")
6. Announce the end of the allotted time in a neutral, tactful way. ("We'll have to stop now because of the time. Let's set up your next appointment up front.") Be careful not to attribute the end of an interview to other waiting patients, to lunch, or to your going home to your family, any of which could suggest to patients that they are less important than other concerns.
7. Observe a valued colleague or instructor during a patient interview, and time the different sections of the interview. Often, you may be surprised at how much information can be obtained with a few questions and much listening.
8. Observe your own interviews by audiotaping or videotaping, with the patient's permission. Time the period before the first interruption, the time spent talking versus listening, and the overall length of the interview portion of the appointment.

In their clerkship rotations, most students learn different forms of clinical interviews for different specialties. A routine prenatal appointment is structured much differently and uses time differently than an emergency room visit. Despite the differences in total time with patients and data obtained, *all* effective interviews share a common structure: They all start with open-ended questions followed by attentive listening. The clinician then focuses inquiries, asks routine questions, and keeps an eye on the clock to avoid a rushed ending.

A 1995 survey of both patients and doctors assessed the perception of how much time doctors spent with their patients. The survey found that patients felt the time together was inadequate four times more often than the doctors felt this (6). It is unlikely that the typical busy physician's schedule will change to allow for more time with individual patients. What can change, however, is different use of limited time. With open-ended questions and allowing patients to describe their agenda in the first two minutes, physicians can maximize the results of limited time and improve patient satisfaction, as well as improve diagnostic accuracy and medical outcomes.

KEY POINTS

1. Time management is the physician's responsibility.
2. Early interruptions have multiple negative effects on the interview.
3. Time management techniques include tracking the time with notes, placing clocks in strategic places, and giving patients "five-minute warnings."
4. Video- or audiotaping interviews allows for direct feedback on time management.

REFERENCES

1. Beckman HB, Frankel RM. The effect of physician behavior on the collection of data. Ann Intern Med 1984;101:692–696.
2. Marvel MK, Epstein RM, Flowers K, Beckman HB. Soliciting the patient's agenda: have we improved? JAMA 1999;281: 283–287.
3. Britten N, Stevenson FA, Barry CA, et al. Misunderstandings in prescribing decisions in general practice: qualitative study. BMJ 2000;320:484–488.
4. Stewart MA, McWhinney IR, Buck CW. The doctor/patient relationship and its effect upon outcome. J R Coll Gen Pract 1979;29:77–81.
5. Stewart MA Effective physician–patient communication and health outcomes: a review. Can Med Assoc J 1995;152:1423–1433.
6. Worthlin Group. Communication and the physician/patient relationship: a physician and consumer communication survey. West Haven, CT: Bayer Institute for Health Care Communication, 1995.

4

Engage

"Engagement" is the first of the four "E's" in the model for clinical communication, as developed by Keller and Carroll (1) and expanded by the Bayer Institute (2). This model describes specific behaviors and skills that are practical and "doable" for clinicians at all levels, from the beginner to the experienced practitioner. This model's approach is particularly helpful because it gives specific guidelines for communication skills and does not depend on any theoretical base. The four E's are Engage, Empathize, Educate, and Enlist.

The first thing any clinician does when he or she meets with another person is to *engage* with that person. The better the engagement or the connection, the better the communication. Positive engagement leads to partnership, a feeling that the doctor and the patient are working together in ways that are rewarding to the doctor and beneficial to the patient (1, 2). Sometimes patients engage negatively with their doctors with angry complaints or "refusal to get better" (addressed in Chapter 9), but most patients are willing partners in positive engagement. They highly value a partnership feeling with their doctors and rate good communication as the most important part of it (3). Engagement is the first step to building the type of therapeutic relationship that gives doctors their power to heal.

There are a number of potential barriers to a positive engagement. A common problem is the "high control"

CLINICAL VIGNETTE 4.1

Dr. Jones is a busy third-year resident in internal medicine. He was on call last night and is now seeing patients in his "continuing care" clinic. Ms. Sumner is a new patient who is transferring from her previous doctor because of a change in insurance. She has high blood pressure and her mother recently had a devastating stroke.

Doctor Jones enters the room with the chart in hand. He begins to speak to his patient while glancing at the information written by the screening nurse.

Dr. Jones: Good morning, Ms. Sumner, I see you are here to have your blood pressure monitored and that you are on Atenolol and that your pressure is 135/90 today. That seems like pretty good control to me.

Ms. Sumner: Well, yes, I guess.

Dr. Jones: Let me check your heart and lungs to make sure you don't have any other problems. You are otherwise healthy, right?

Ms. Sumner: I guess so.

Dr. Jones: (Listens to her heart and lungs.) No past surgeries, hospitalizations, major medical problems . . .

Ms. Sumner: No.

Dr. Jones: No use of tobacco, drugs, or alcohol . . .

Ms. Sumner: No, nothing like that.

Dr. Jones: Well great. Let's just continue your Atenolol, and I will see you again in 6 or 12 months. Any questions?

Ms. Sumner: I guess not.

Dr. Jones: Great. Nice meeting you. (He exits, feeling relieved that he now has one less patient to see before he can go home to sleep.)

Ms. Sumner: Goodbye, Doctor. (She sits on the examining table in the paper gown, missing her previous doctor very much.)

interviewing style (see Vignette 4.1). This is the clinician who interprets the role of doctor as that of the busy technical expert who cannot be expected to ask about feelings or who does not allow patients to tell their story in their own words. Effective communication does not imply that all physicians will become "therapists." Instead, effective communication allows the physician to do his or her core job—treating medical problems—as effectively as possible. The added benefits from good communication are improved relationships with patients and increased job satisfaction.

With his high control interview style, Dr. Jones in our example loses the chance to positively engage his patient and to build an effective patient–doctor relationship. In the interest of efficiency, he has sacrificed his most powerful healing tool—a relationship with his patient. Possible consequences are poor patient adherence—Ms. Sumner may miss follow-up appointments or stop taking the medication as prescribed.

The strategies for positively engaging a patient are not mysterious or complicated. They include joining, eliciting the agenda, and setting the agenda.

JOINING

Joining occurs in the first part of any visit, with the first words out of your mouth. A "welcome" or "glad to see you" accompanied with a smile and eye contact sets the tone of warmth and welcome (1). A doctor's use of time during the first few minutes and the type of questions asked (see Chapter 3) have a large impact on how well he or she engages with a patient. Nonverbal communication is particularly important in the first moments of meeting. Making eye contact at the same time as shaking someone's hand is a powerful, positive welcoming gesture.

In the example of Vignette 4.2, Dr. White laid the foundation for positive engagement. He approached a somewhat difficult to engage patient with warmth, friendliness,

CLINICAL VIGNETTE 4.2

Dr. White is a family medicine doctor who schedules new patients on Mondays. Today, he sees Mrs. Schmidt, an elderly widow who has recently moved to the area to be closer to her children and grandchildren.

Dr. White: Mrs. Schmidt, welcome. (He takes her hand, smiles, and looks at her. The chart is laid on the counter.) I am Dr. White, one of the doctors in this group. How are you today?

Mrs. Schmidt: Fair to middlin', as they say.

Dr. White: OK, "fair to middlin'." What can I do for you today?

Mrs. Schmidt: Nothing much. My daughter wanted me to come in and see a doctor.

Dr. White: How about you? What are you wanting today?

Mrs. Schmidt: Doctor, I don't know which end is up. I just moved here from California, half my life is still in packing crates, and I'm just trying to keep my family happy by coming to this appointment.

Dr. White: Hmm. Sounds like there is a lot going on. Let me propose this. Since you are here today, let's review you past medical treatments, do a physical exam, look at any current medical concerns you have, and in the meantime I'll get to know a little more about you and how I can be most helpful. What do you think? Sound like a plan?

Mrs. Schmidt: That sounds like a plan.

and flexibility. He recognized her ambivalence in being in his office and offered her increased participation in planning.

An important aspect of joining is communicating to patients that you are interested and curious about them as people, not just as a medical diagnosis (1). The best way to show this interest is to ask about something unrelated to their medical problems (see Box 4.1).

BOX 4.1
Examples of Engagement Questions

For new patients:

Before we start on your medical history, I'd like to know a little more about you. Where you work, what you do for fun, those sorts of things.

It's nice to meet you. When I meet new patients I like to start off understanding a bit about them. I can see from the badge on your shirt that you work with horses. Are you a rider?

Hi, Ms. Lake. I'm Doctor Greenfeld. How are you today?

You moved here recently from Kentucky? How has the transition to New England been for you and your family?

For returning patients:

How is that new grandbaby? Is she sitting up yet?

How was spring break? Did you go on a trip?

Any luck selling your house/getting that promotion/getting your seedlings covered before the frost?

Some students and doctors feel uncomfortable asking about "personal" matters. However, the non-medical details are what make a patient a person and allow doctors to have a richer understanding of their patients' lives. On occasion, patients will find these types of inquiries intrusive and will give clear messages for a doctor to back off by responding minimally or not at all to non-medical questions. Yet almost all patients value being seen and known to their doctor as a person.

Different engagement strategies will work better with certain patient populations. Some patients who present particular challenges (such as angry patients) are discussed in Chapter 9.

Young Children: (see Vignette 4.3) Physicians who are also parents have an advantage in working with young children because they have background experience in what a child is interested in at different developmental stages. Often, the parent of a young patient can offer some hints

CLINICAL VIGNETTE 4.3

MD: (sits on floor or squatting to be at 3-year-old child's eye level) Hey there, Sara. I'm Doctor Bill.
Sara: (is silent, without eye contact)
MD: I bet you are a Winnie the Pooh fan. I see you have Pooh Bear on your hat. Who do like best—Pooh, Tigger, or Rabbit?
Sara: Tigger.
MD: What do you like about Tigger?
Sara: He jumps!
MD: Wow! He does! Do you jump?
Sara: I jump on Poppa's chair!
MD: Great! What else do you do?
Sara: I jump on the couch!
MD: All right, Jumping Sara! Your mommy told me you have a sore throat and a cough. I want to check these out so you can feel better. Will you jump onto the table for me?

about what the child is interested in. This allows for engaging the child at his or her level.

Adolescents: (see Vignette 4.4) It is developmentally appropriate for adolescents to be wary of authority figures and to be immersed in a peer culture that values music and clothing as means of asserting independence and individuality. Similar to the approach to the young child, touching down on a topic at the adolescent's level is helpful in engagement. Although there is wide variation of personality types and styles, most adolescents are concerned about privacy and autonomy, so early discussion of these topics can help engage a patient.

Elderly Patients: (see Vignette 4.5) Older people have a variety of special concerns and needs. For some, the visit to the physician's office provides an important source of social contact. For other elderly patients, physical limita-

CLINICAL VIGNETTE 4.4

MD: Hi. I'm Dr. Brown. You are Jacob? What would you like for me to call you?
Jake: Jake.
MD: All right Jake, good to meet you. Before we get started here, I want to let you know that what we talk about can be private from your parents, which is why they are in the waiting room now. The only things they can hear about are the things you say are OK to tell them or the things they need to know to consent to medical treatment. There are some exceptions to this—life and death things—and we'll talk about this again if those sorts of things come up. Any questions about that?
Jake: No.
MD: OK. I'd like to start off by learning about things you like. What do you like to do after school?
Jake: I don't know. (pauses) Skateboard. Video games.
MD: What video games do you like?
Jake: All sorts.
MD: Tomb Raider?
Jake: Yeah, that one's all right.
MD: Did you see the movie?
Jake: Yeah, about four times.
MD: Must have been a pretty good movie!
Jake: Yeah.

tions require special attention to the interview setting—such as providing chairs with back and arm support for those who have a hard time rising.

Health Care Professionals: (see Vignette 4.6) When physicians treat other health care professionals, they are sometimes uncomfortable having a dual role with a colleague. As a result, there is sometimes a tendency to minimize the patient care aspect of the visit and spend a disproportionate amount of time on professional small talk.

CLINICAL VIGNETTE 4.5

MD: Hello, Mrs. James—how are you today?
Mrs. James: I'm all right, Doctor.
MD: Before we get started, I'd like to check on a couple of things. Can you hear me OK, and are you comfortable?
Mrs. James: I can hear you all right. I'm comfortable.
MD: Good. And how are things at Crestview Manor?
Mrs. James: Well, the food's no good. But the people are nice. And my little dog gets to stay with me.
MD: How is Pepper?
Mrs. James: Oh, he's good. You know, he's a funny little dog. He loves to eat mashed potatoes.

CLINICAL VIGNETTE 4.6

MD: Hello, Doctor!
Patient: Hello, Doctor!
MD: How goes the world of pediatric pulmonology?
Patient: Good. Lots of new developments in pediatric asthma. It's like having new weapons in an old war.
MD: Sounds interesting. Now let's get to you. How have you been feeling lately?

Although this may decrease the discomfort level, it does not provide the patient with the same level of care granted to nonprofessionals.

Neurologically Impaired Patients: (see Vignette 4.7) Patients who are neurologically impaired or developmentally disabled need the same respect and consideration as unimpaired people. At times, the physician and the caregiver may discuss the patient in the third person and may even forget the patient is present and listening. Even though

CLINICAL VIGNETTE 4.7

MD: Hello, Mr. Jones, Mrs. Jones. How are you today, sir?
Mr. Jones: (is aphasic, cannot answer in words but nods head up and down)
MD: Does your nodding mean "OK"?
Mr. Jones: (nods again)
MD: Good. Today I will be asking your wife some things like how your speech and physical therapy have been going. If we start to talk about something and you disagree or want to add something, can you give a wave?
Mr. Jones: (nods again)
MD: Good—that way we will know to check with you on it too.

a neurologically impaired individual may not be able to follow everything that is being said, he or she can often extract information about others' feelings by observing facial expressions and emotional overtones in speech.

Another way to effectively engage with patients is to show interest in the words they use to describe medical problems and adapt the physician's own vocabulary a bit to reflect the patient's use of language (1, 2) (see Box 4.2).

BOX 4.2
Adapting to the Patient's Language

What was it about the food that made you have a *spell*?

How big was this *teeny-weeny* scrape?

You mentioned a *five-alarm* headache. What did you do for that?

Who else in your family has *high blood*? Is there another word the doctor has used to describe this problem?

At the time of your husband's *nervous breakdown,* what medications was he taking?

I understand that you don't like the new *sugar pill* because it gives you a *tinny* taste in your mouth.

When the physician uses the patient's language, it is important that he or she is confident about exactly what the patient means. The phrase "sugar pill," for example, sometimes refers to oral hypoglycemics but might be describing a placebo pill. After clarifying, the doctor can document in the chart the more accurate medical term and continue to use the patient's words in the interview whenever it feels appropriate.

ELICITING AND SETTING THE AGENDA

In addition to communicating friendly interest in the patient, another task of engagement is to establish the agenda at the beginning of each interview (1). Medical students are taught to obtain and document the "chief complaint." Almost no patients, however, arrive at their doctor's visit with a single, well-articulated problem. Patients usually have a story about their problems and have a list of concerns that includes several medical issues and a few psychosocial problems as well. One research study found that the average patient had five problems they wanted to discuss at an office visit, but only rarely did a patient actually communicate the full list of problems (their "agenda") to the doctor. The agenda items that were not mentioned led to more misunderstandings and problems (4). Clearly, it is in the patient's best interest to tell the doctor about all of the problems on their "list." Most patients, however, need some help in effectively communicating their agenda.

The best way to help patients communicate their agenda is to ask open-ended questions. These are questions that require more than a yes/no or other one-word answer (1) (see Box 4.3).

Open-ended questions almost always convey an interest in the patient and do not guide the patient into answering a certain way. These types of questions invite patients to tell their "story" and to relate their full agenda. Students and doctors often worry that they will lose control

BOX 4.3
Open-ended Questions

What problems would you like to discuss today?

What else?

Can you help me understand that better?

Describe for me what was going on for you.

Tell me more about that.

How are you feeling?

What do you think of the new medication?

It's been a whole year since I last saw you—how have things been?

of the interview with open-ended questions—there is a fear that these questions can lead to endless responses without ever getting to key medical information. Doctors become impatient, as patience is a skill seldom taught in medical school. The bottom line, however, is effectiveness. Effective doctors elicit the story and the agenda, and research shows that this does not take much, if any, extra time (5, 6). Chapter 3 gives examples of ways to use open-ended questions and stay in control of the time.

An important part of hearing the patient's story is *showing* that it is heard. Both verbally and nonverbally (by leaning forward and having an interested facial expression), the doctor shows that he or she hears both the facts of

BOX 4.4
Ways of Acknowledging the Story

It sounds like your breathing was causing you so much trouble that you canceled your trip to the high school reunion.

Mrs. Miller, from what you have told me, the new medication helps your sleep but makes you feel too "hung over" in the morning.

Your description of your cough helps me understand why you decided to stop the over-the-counter cough syrup and come in today.

CLINICAL VIGNETTE 4.8

Acknowledging the Story

Mr. Jaeger made an appointment to see his general practitioner because of left leg pain. He is secretly fearful of being shamed by the doctor because of a "trivial" complaint. He is also fearful that the pain could be due to some major problem like cancer. He describes his pain to his doctor—steady pain during the day, worsening at night, slowly progressing to the point where he has difficulty walking up stairs.

His doctor replies, "Mr. Jaeger, from what you have told me, your pain is getting worse and is starting to really get in the way of your daily routine. It's concerning to you and to me, and I'm glad you came in today so we can check it out."

the problems and the associated feelings (2) (see Box 4.4). Using the patient's language as described above also gives the patient the message that the doctor was really listening. A brief physician summary acknowledges the story and allows for any corrections.

The doctor should be aware that a patient's medical problems and concerns usually carry an emotional element (see Vignette 4.8). Identifying and validating these emotions are a key part of empathy, which can be a part of the engagement process (see Chapter 5).

In addition to using open-ended questions and acknowledging the story, which give the patient the opportunity to mention a number of concerns, doctors can prompt patients to give a more complete agenda, including psychosocial problems. Most people feel a bit shy bringing up mood problems or sexual problems. The physician can make it clear that he or she is interested in *all* of the patient's problems (see Box 4.5). All of the identified problems can be part of the patient's "problem list," which is a work-

BOX 4.5
Eliciting the Agenda

I'm glad to hear that rash has cleared up. How are other things going for you?

Sometimes when someone has diabetes, it affects other parts of their life such as mood or sexual functioning. Do you have any concerns about mood, such as depression, or about sex, such as your sexual response?

We've spent a good deal of time reviewing your blood pressure meds over the last few visits. Before we look at that today, I'd like to ask whether you have anything else you would like to bring up.

You hinted at some problems you were having with your son's illness. Would you like to discuss that today?

ing list that allows the doctor to track the different medical problems and concerns over time (2).

The physician who is effective in joining with the patient and eliciting the agenda, is likely to be in the position of having identified more problems than can realistically be addressed in the scheduled appointment time. This makes it necessary for the doctor to further develop a partnership with the patient and negotiate or agree upon the agenda for that visit (see Box 4.6). Emergency problems usually do not require any discussion, but a combination of new and old problems makes it necessary at the beginning to ask the patient questions to clarify expectations for that visit (1, 2) (see Vignette 4.9).

Both patients and doctors are more satisfied with the time spent together during an appointment when they have

BOX 4.6
Clarifying the Agenda

What are you hoping we will accomplish today?

You mentioned a few concerns—which is most important for us to address today?

How would you like to use today's appointment time?

(adapted from Refs. 1 & 2)

CLINICAL VIGNETTE 4.9

Clarifying the Agenda

Dr. Fischer has Mrs. Billings scheduled for an appointment to follow up on a previous visit when she presented with a new onset headache. The doctor starts the appointment with an open-ended question ("How are things since I saw you last?") and is a bit surprised with the patient's reply.

Mrs. Billings: Well, Doctor, I'm sorry to say that the headache is not at all better, even though I've been taking the Motrin® as you said and I even cut out red wine at dinner. I think it would be a good thing for me to get a brain scan or something. I also am having pain in my stomach now, with nausea whenever I'm a passenger in a car. And out of the blue, my sleep has gotten worse.

Dr. Fischer: It sounds like there are a couple of new problems. Anything else?

Mrs. Billings: Well, I was reluctant to mention this, but I'm just so damned irritable, I'm wondering if it's change of life.

Dr. Fischer: That's another important issue. Our scheduled time today limits us to focus on one of the four things: headache, stomach pain, sleep, or possible change of life symptoms. Which do *you* feel is most important today, and which can wait until we are able to reschedule our next appointment?

Mrs. Billings: Let's get this headache under control. Maybe it's the stress of thinking I have a brain tumor that's upsetting my stomach and my sleep. I can come back later, no problem.

Dr. Fischer: OK, let's review the next step in evaluating your headache.

engaged positively, identified a complete agenda, and have directly discussed how they will use the available time.

KEY POINTS

1. Engaging a patient begins with greeting the patient as a person.
2. Different types of engagement techniques can work for different types of patients.
3. Patients often have multiple problems or agendas and need help stating them.
4. Physicians and patients can negotiate at the beginning of an appointment how time will be used.

REFERENCES

1. Keller VF, Carroll JG. A new model for physician–patient communication. Patient Educ Couns 1994;23:134–140.
2. Bayer Institute for Health Care Communication. Clinician–patient communication to enhance health outcomes: a workshop manual. West Haven, CT: Bayer Institute, 1998.
3. Worthlin Group. Communication and the physician/patient relationship: a physician and consumer communication survey. West Haven, CT: Bayer Institute for Health Care Communication, 1995.
4. Barry CA, Bradley CP, Britten N, et al. Patient's unvoiced agendas in general practice consultations: qualitative study. BMJ 2000;320:1246–1250.
5. Levinson W, Roter DL, Mullooly JP, et al. Physician–patient communication: the relationship with malpractice claims among primary care physicians and surgeons. JAMA 1997;277:553–559.
6. Marvel MK, Doherty WJ, Weiner E. Medical interviewing by exemplary family physicians. J Fam Pract 1998;47:343–348.

5

Empathize

Empathy, the second "E," is such an important element in doctor–patient communications that this section starts with a definition: Empathy is understanding and participating in another person's feeling state—sharing their emotional experience. It is different from sympathy, which describes the listener's feelings, but not an understanding or sharing of the pa-tient's emotions (see Vignettes 5.1 and 5.2).

Whenever a patient brings in a medical problem, he or she brings in feelings about that problem as well. If the doctor can identify the patient's feelings, and then show acknowledgment and acceptance, the patient will have received a powerful "medicine" in the form of empathy. Empathy can be hard work, and most doctors' empathic skills develop with practice over the course of years. Studies of doctors and therapists have shown that empathy, and the resulting therapeutic alliance, are critical factors in overall medical outcome (1). In fact, a placebo in the hands of a very empathic clinician was as effective as an active antidepressant medication with less effective clinicians in a double-blinded study of depression (2). Patients in a 1995 survey rated the item "Physician understands you" higher than any other communication factor in importance for the physician–patient relationship (3). We are fortunate that such a powerful tool is available to all students and practitioners of medicine. Although some individuals come to their training with more natural empathy, empathic

CLINICAL VIGNETTE 5.1

Empathy versus Sympathy 1
Mr. Xavier, who is 57, comes to his doctor's office for a follow-up appointment after a lower GI endoscopy. The results of the exam were normal, but his doctor can't help but notice that he looks sad and drawn. When this is mentioned, the patient tells his doctor that his small business is failing because of competition from the big chain stores and that he must either close his store now or watch it go into bankruptcy.
Sympathetic reply: "I'm sorry to hear that is happening. It is a sad story." (The patient feels that the doctor is a nice person.)
Empathic reply: "What a huge loss for you—after years of building it up and now seeing it end like this . . ." (The patient feels that the doctor truly "gets it," that he understands and shares in his feelings about the current problems and losses.)

behavior toward patients is made up of very learnable skills (4).

The first part of having and showing empathy is seeing and hearing patients and letting them know they have been seen and heard. The second part, which is more challenging for most doctors but is also learnable, involves letting a patient know that he or she is accepted as a person (5).

SEEING AND HEARING THE PATIENT

There are a number of practical steps doctors can take to increase their empathic response to a patient. The first is to identify and remove barriers to seeing and hearing the patient. In every medical setting there are potential

CLINICAL VIGNETTE 5.2

Empathy versus Sympathy 2
Mrs. Lovett, 62, has had a number of skin cancers on her nose, forehead, and cheeks recently removed. The scars are well healed but have left hypopigmented indentations in each area where a cancer was removed. She is embarrassed by these marks and asks her doctor during a follow-up appointment about what can be done. Unfortunately, the doctor tells her, only cosmetic make-up is possible.
Sympathetic reply: "It's too bad we can't patch you up a little better. The scars are better than the cancer, though." (Mrs. Lovett feels sad and a bit ashamed for having asked her doctor about the scars.)
Empathic reply: "I can tell by what you've said that the scars are very noticeable and embarrassing to you. I wish there was more I could do—I can see how disappointed you are." (Mrs. Lovett feels the doctor has understood her, and this, at least, soothes her sadness. Her doctor can't fix the scars, but he wishes he could and he understands her disappointment.)

barriers—the most common is the medical chart. Simply lowering the chart onto the lap or table during the first part of the interview and setting it aside at appropriate time opens up the opportunity for the doctor to be more "present" with the patient. Doctors should avoid sitting at a desk that comes between them and the patient; chairs on a diagonal are less likely to make the patient feel "cut off" from the doctor who is talking and listening to them (4). In a hospital room, doctors can sit at eye level to the patient and pull the chair up closer to the bed. Hovering over a patient can give the impression that the doctor is talking to, not with, someone. By sitting in a chair,

CLINICAL VIGNETTE 5.3

"Mr. Johnson, I want to make sure I get all of the information as you tell it, so please forgive me for taking notes as we go."

the doctor also communicates his or her willingness to be there for at least a few minutes. Empathic doctors make eye contact when they ask questions and when the patient is speaking. They minimize their writing in front of the patient whenever possible. If they need to take many notes, they apologize in advance to the patient (4) as in Vignette 5.3.

Although it is not usually socially acceptable to make observations or comments on other people's feelings unless they are close friends or family, in the medical interview, recognizing and acknowledging the patient's feeling state is such an important skill that it should be taught routinely in all medical schools. Sometimes patients volunteer what they are experiencing emotionally, but more often they are not so direct. Instead, the doctor has to pick up on patient clues. Recognizing the clues to underlying emotions in a patient is a critical step in communicating empathy (6, 7) (see Box 5.1).

Often, these are new skills that the student must learn outside of the medical school curriculum. Sometimes doctors interrupt patients or change the subject when patients bring up potentially emotional topics, because doctors are uncomfortable with the possibility of an emotional expression such as tears or anger (6). It might feel intrusive or awkward to specifically address facial expressions, tone of voice, or statements of emotion, but these observations are exactly what communicates empathy. With practice, observing and inviting patients to talk about their emotions can become second nature, and one of the most rewarding parts of patient care.

BOX 5.1
Observing the Patient's Emotional State

Dr. Kellogg has been describing the recommended course of treatment for a patient with prostate cancer. She notices that when she says "radiation," Mr. Williams' face blanches and he looks at the floor.
Dr. Kellogg: "You looked a bit troubled when I mentioned radiation just now. Let's talk a bit about that."

Dr. Little is discussing the routine repair of a colostomy with his patient when she bursts into tears.
Dr. Little: "Where are those tears coming from? Let's talk about what is upsetting to you."

Dr. Smythe is talking to her patient Ms. Laub, a 19-year-old college student. Avoiding eye contact with the doctor, Ms. Laub cooly relates how, in the waiting room, she overheard the nurse behind the counter say, rather loudly, "Another college student, probably here for either birth control or a yeast infection."
Dr. Smythe: "I'm sorry that happened—my guess is that it is really upsetting or embarrassing when your privacy is not respected, and you might feel angry about it now."

When one asks for, observes, and acknowledges patients' feelings and values, they know they truly have been seen and heard. Another important way to communicate such acknowledgment is through nonverbal facial expressions and gestures. At times, leaning forward and showing an understanding of sadness through a softened facial expression can communicate understanding of a patient's feelings better than words. A light touch—to the back of a patient's hand or shoulder—during an emotionally difficult time is also experienced by most patients as a powerful empathic gesture. A touch or eye contact that lasts only three seconds can better provide connection and shared experience than a paragraph of words. Other times it is most appropriate, and empathic, for the doctor to allow a patient to simply ventilate his or her anger and grief and to give noncommittal nods, accompanied by facilitating comments such as "Right, right," "Of course," or "I see."

ACCEPTANCE

The core of empathy is acceptance. After patients have experienced being seen and heard by their doctor, they need to feel that the doctor accepts them as well (5). A term sometimes used is "unconditional positive regard." This suggests that the doctor cares for patients even if they are frightened, poor, angry, noncompliant with the prescription, disfigured, addicted to drugs, or if their illness gets worse rather than better. Empathy naturally brings forth compassion and is a skill of nonjudgment. For some students, this skill is a formidable challenge, and they have difficulty in not judging a patient because of core beliefs and attitudes acquired prior to medical school (8). For these students, it is important to find a role model—a doctor or colleague who both speaks and acts in ways that demonstrate a loving tolerance and compassion for others (see Vignette 5.4).

CLINICAL VIGNETTE 5.4

A third-year medical student was assigned to a busy labor and delivery unit in an inner-city hospital. Many of the patients were teenage mothers, and some were in early labor due to crack cocaine use or opiate withdrawal.

One young patient was in a great deal of discomfort during active labor. She was hot and sweaty and had begun to retch. The medical student called for her supervisor to find out what to do about the patient's vomiting.

The supervisor wet a washcloth with cool water and placed it on the back of the patient's neck. She smoothed the patient's hair from her face, made eye contact, and told her, "This is the hard part . . . It will get better after a little while. You are doing a great job."

BARRIERS TO EMPATHY

There are a number of potential barriers to a doctor developing a healthy empathy for patients. Some of the barriers reside in the patient, others in the doctors. Often the way students and residents are trained—long clinical hours and apparent disregard to personal needs—creates a culture that neglects feelings and discourages humanism.

Some patients are "empathically challenging" to their doctors. A way to increase compassion and understanding for such a patient is to find something about the patient that is likable. This could be a taste in clothes or literature, or a personality trait such as persistence or dignity. Identifying at least one likable trait may allow for friendlier feelings for that person and enhance the doctor's empathic response.

Some students of empathy dig deeper into the reasons why we can empathize and identify with people so different from ourselves. They find that humans are more alike than different. Regardless of which side of the chart or the bed-rails they sit, both people in the doctor–patient relationship share fundamentals of the human experience. Everyone is born into a family. Everyone has hopes and fears and disappointments. Everyone wishes to avoid unpleasant medical tests and treatments. No one ever wants to be seriously ill or disabled, but everyone is at some risk for cancer or depression or being hit by a bus. These similarities come into sharp relief whenever a doctor tends to a patient who is also a physician and realizes that being a doctor does not magically protect anyone from tragedy or illness.

Certain types of patients evoke different responses for different individuals. For some doctors, working with small children brings out unreserved empathic feelings. For others, working with elderly patients elicits the doctor's most genuine emotional connections. At times, a certain type of patient can awaken in the doctor feelings of irritation, contempt, or guilt. These negative feelings can lead to an emotional retreat and an empathic "lapse," or failure, on the part of the doctor.

In addition to the particular challenges a patient might present to almost every doctor, there are individual variations among the doctors as well. Novack and colleagues describe how a physician's negative response to a patient (or a type of patient) can reflect the physician's unrecognized feelings and attitudes. Personal awareness on the part of the physician can improve relationships with patients (8, 9). Chapter 9 addresses a number of difficult patient scenarios.

If a student or doctor struggles with responding empathetically to a patient, he or she would probably benefit from discussing this with a trusted colleague or supervisor who could offer some objective observations about both the student and the patient(s), as well as offer suggestions about the problem (see Vignette 5.5).

For example, a student's negative feelings toward a patient may lead to his avoiding and rejecting the patient. A supervisor might ask the student if he had had any particular experiences with patients like this in the past that could be coloring his response to this patient. Sometimes peers are wonderful empathy consultants—they can confront a colleague's empathic weaknesses in gentle or even humorous ways.

COMPASSION

Compassion is empathy in action. With an empathic understanding of a patient, most physicians behave in ways to decrease the patient's suffering. At times, this is an offer of support for a patient's past actions or an action on the part of the physician that "goes the extra mile."

Offering support for a patient's past actions does not imply approval of their behavior or decisions. It is merely an understanding and acceptance of them (10) (see Vignettes 5.6 and 5.7).

CLINICAL VIGNETTE 5.5

Empathy Consultation

James is a fourth-year medical student currently on a neurology elective rotation. He is busy, is on call every third night, and is working with very sick patients, including head trauma patients. One of his patients is under arrest for suspected gang violence and is handcuffed to the bed, with a deputy sheriff sitting outside of the door. James complains to his supervisor that this patient shouldn't be taking up a hospital bed but should be in jail.

Supervisor: James, I can see that you are tired and frustrated. Let's take a few minutes and look at this patient. You are the medical student and here is your patient, probably both a victim and a perpetrator of gang violence. What do you think might be going on in his head right now?

James: Well, he is probably hurting from the head injury and the stitches.

Supervisor: What else?

James: Well, maybe he's worried about what's going to happen with him, going to jail.

Supervisor: What else?

James: I saw his mother in there yesterday, crying. He probably feels bad about that too.

Supervisor: How can we show him that we understand at least a little bit of what is going on in his life right now?

James: I guess I could ask him how the pain is and what worries he has.

Supervisor: That would involve spending some time with this man.

James: And actually talking to him.

CLINICAL VIGNETTE 5.6

Support of Past Actions 1
Patient: I'm sort of embarrassed I let that lump get so big before I came in. I actually noticed it about six months ago, and it wasn't until it hurt so much I couldn't sleep that I called for an appointment. I hope it isn't anything serious. I hate dealing with medical problems.
MD: You know, it's really human nature to try and avoid unpleasant things and I think we all secretly wish lumps and pains will just go away. And sometimes we try and wait them out. So I understand why you waited six months. Our job now is to deal with it, especially because it's getting bigger and more painful.

Support of Past Actions 2
Patient: I know now it was the wrong thing to do, but I thought maybe the pills were making me sick so I stopped them. I didn't know my blood pressure would go up so high.
MD: Maybe stopping the medication was the only decision that made sense to you at the time. Let's review your blood pressures and talk about another medicine, as well as the best plan of action if you have side effects in the future.

KEY POINTS

1. Empathy, the sharing of another's emotional state, is a powerful tool in building rapport and improving medical outcomes.
2. Most patients give hints about their emotions during a visit, rather than direct statements. Physicians with empathic skills recognize the hints and help the patient to fully describe the underlying emotions.
3. Barriers to empathy are many, and all can be effectively overcome.

CLINICAL VIGNETTE 5.7

"Going the Extra Mile" 1

Patient: I hope you don't mind. My parents were visiting and they are so worried about my illness that I was hoping you could spend a few moments with them. I know you are awful busy . . . they are in the waiting room.

MD: Bring them right in, I'd like to meet them. . . . Hello, Mr. and Mrs. Phillips. I'm Dr. Henry. I'm glad you could come in today. I know as a parent myself that even when our kids are grown up they are still our kids and we worry about them. How can I be helpful to you today?

"Going the Extra Mile" 2

Patient: I blew it. You gave me the name of the orthopedic surgeon I was supposed to see, but I got so busy taking care of my mother and getting my father into a nursing home that I lost it, and now it's three weeks later and I should be scheduled for surgery and I don't know what to do. I can't believe how bad my foot hurts.

MD: It's too bad that didn't work out better—it sounds like you've been working hard to take good care of your parents. I can try and call the surgeon myself today. I know her pretty well. She may be willing to schedule you in as an emergency appointment. I'll ask you to wait after our appointment, and I'll call her office to see if we can get you in today.

4. Acceptance and support of a patient, as well as compassion, are part of a physician's empathic response.

REFERENCES

1. Squier R. A model of empathic understanding and adherence to treatment regimens in practitioner–patient relationships. Soc Sci Med 1990;30:325–339.

2. Blatt SJ, Sanislow CA, Zuroff DC, Pilkonis PA. Characteristics of effective therapists: further analyses of data from the National Institute of Mental Health Treatment of Depression Collaborative Research Program. J Consult Clin Psychol 1996;64:1276–1284.
3. Worthlin Group. Communication and the physician/patient relationship: a physician and consumer communication survey. West Haven, CT: Bayer Institute for Health Care Communication, 1995.
4. Keller VF, Carroll JG. A new model for physician–patient communication. Patient Educ Couns 1994;23:134–140.
5. Bayer Institute for Health Care Communication. Clinician–patient communication to enhance health outcomes: a workshop manual. West Haven, CT: Bayer Institute, 1998.
6. Suchman AL, Markakis K, Beckamn HB, Frankel R. A model of empathic communication in the medical interview. JAMA 1997;277:678–682.
7. Branch WT, Malik TK. Using "windows of opportunities" in brief interviews to understand patients' concerns. JAMA 1993;269:1667–1668.
8. Novack DH, Suchman AL, Clark W, et al. Calibrating the physician: personal awareness and effective patient care. JAMA 1997;278:502–509.
9. Epstein RM. Mindful practice. JAMA 1999;282:833–839.
10. Platt FW, Keller VF. Empathic communication: a teachable and learnable skill. J Gen Intern Med 1994;9:222–226.

6

Educate

Of the four "E's," the third is "Educate." Patient education techniques complement Engage and Empathize in the effective physician interview. It is critical in improving outcome, because patient education has a dramatic impact on patient adherence to medical treatment (1, 2).

Adherence, sometimes called compliance, is how well a patient follows the prescribed treatment. A patient can have good or poor adherence to medication, diet, exercise, or any other treatment intervention, which then leads to good or bad outcomes. As every physician would expect, a patient's failure to follow medical treatment (such as missing appointments, using medication incorrectly, or not monitoring blood sugar) leads to a failure to improve or maintain health. Studies of the effect of patient education show that brief educational interventions with patients can have dramatic benefits on outcomes such as blood sugar and pain control. Educated patients sometimes need less medication overall (3).

Almost every study examining patient adherence rates has found them to be surprisingly low. For example, medical prescriptions are not taken or are taken incorrectly more than 60% of the time (4). Patients typically do not follow their doctor's recommendations for prescription medications, self-care, or exercise. This chapter highlights the specific education techniques that are associated with better patient adherence.

Patients are always curious about their illnesses. Although they may not ask many questions (due to anxiety and concerns about being "pushy" or using up "too much of the doctor's time"), most patients want more education about their illness than physicians typically give. A recent public service advertisement put out by the National Patient Safety Foundation highlights the need for patient education with this advice for patients: "Speak up if you have questions . . . and don't be shy about asking . . . for more information." The same advertisement recommends that patients understand what a prescription is for and ask about the different options available to them for treatment (5). This advice may surprise many physicians, who believe they are already providing their patients with the necessary information. A study of physician communication found that physicians usually underestimate a patient's desire for information and overestimate the time they actually spend giving information to patients by a factor of *nine.* On average, physicians spent only one minute per visit educating their patients (6).

Assuming patients will ask for the information they need is a dangerous assumption. For example, cancer specialists who wait for the patient to ask for details of their illness end up withholding information from all but the most assertive and organized patient (7).

The topic of patient education is even more important in light of research that shows how much information patients actually remember from their visits with physicians. In a study of patients with chronic illness, roughly only 50% of the patients with diabetes and 35% of patients with hypertension were able to recall information that they had received about reducing alcohol intake or about self-care recommendations regarding diabetic supplies. Predictably, adherence to forgotten information was extremely low, with presumed negative medical outcomes (8).

One obstacle to patient recollection of information may be anxiety during the office visit. Another may be a mismatch of vocabularies. Although most physicians are comfortable using medical terms, most patients do not

BOX 6.1

What do you think is going on with your [blood sugars, pain, bruising, etc.]?

What information do you already have about [foot checks, use of this medication, cardiac rehabilitation]? What else do you want to know at this time?

Sometimes we use the word(s) [depression, stroke, nervous breakdown, high blood] in different ways. What does it mean to you?

understand them and may not ask for clarification. A study of patient understanding of common medical terms found that only 36% of patients could correctly identify the definitions for words such as "depression" and "stroke" (9).

In view of these obstacles and with the firm understanding that patients need to understand their illness and treatment to follow their physician's prescriptions, the education of patients is a critical communication skill. The first step in education is to find out what the patient already knows—some of which could be misinformation (2) (see Box 6.1). Related to a patient's knowledge are his or her beliefs about what is happening. In seeking the patient's level of understanding, it is important to preface questions with a statement such as "I have some ideas about the problems, but first I'd like to ask you . . ." With these words, patients can feel reassured that *they* are not being asked to make the diagnosis. A physician also should elicit a patient's understanding about his or her illness.

The next step in education is to directly address the unspoken but important questions most patients bring to the medical office visit. These questions are especially meaningful with new patients or when the illness is new or puzzling.

1. What has happened to me?
2. Why has this happened?
3. What is going to happen next? What will eventually happen? (1, 2)

CLINICAL VIGNETTE 6.1

"Mr. Jones, I've found that most people are curious about the symptoms they are having. In your case, I think your cough and fever are from bronchitis, which is an inflammation of the large breathing tubes in the lungs. This is most likely caused by infection from bacteria, which is why we treat it with antibiotics. Smoking makes it more likely you would get this, but with antibiotic treatment and overall good rest and nutrition, it is unlikely it will become anything worse than bronchitis and should get better by the end of the week."

"Ms. Green, I know you must be wondering about the easy bruising that you've developed. At this point, I can't be sure about what the problem is, but I want to order some blood tests that should give us quite a bit more of information. I'll call you if there is anything that I think we need to talk about. Otherwise, we can review the tests at our next visit."

These questions represent every patient's desire to know about the diagnosis, cause, and prognosis of their illness (1, 2). Every new patient or established patient with a new problem truly wants to have these questions answered during the course of a visit. Physicians can usually meet the patient's unspoken requests in a straightforward way, using the most simple and most honest response possible. This is particularly true when the physician does not know all the answers. Honest uncertainty is an important fact of everyday physician communication (see Vignette 6.1).

A special area is a patient's unspoken concern that he or she has a very serious problem such as a cancer. Many patients have other unspoken fears, sometimes related to illnesses they have seen in family or friends. If the physician knows about the patient's experiences, he or she can anticipate some of these specific worries (see Vignette 6.2).

CLINICAL VIGNETTE 6.2

"Well, Mrs. Gonzales, I think we are close to understanding your stomach pain. First, let me tell you that it does not appear to be any kind of cancer, which I think you might have been worried about after your mother's recent illness. At this time, the exam and tests lead me to think it is a condition called 'esophageal reflux.' (Here, let me write that down for you.) What that means is that the esophagus, the food tube between your mouth and stomach, is getting reflux or 'backwash' from the acid in the stomach. The acid irritates the sensitive lining of that food tube and can cause a lot of pain, especially after eating certain kinds of foods."

The world of medicine has become increasingly foreign to non-medical people, so patients are likely to have additional unspoken questions that can effectively be addressed as part of patient education. Medical centers are large, bewildering places, and the technological advances that have helped improve health care have added more layers of mystery to the typical patient's medical experiences. Thus, patients often wonder:

1. What are you doing to me?
2. Why are you doing this and not something else?
3. Will it hurt? How long will it take?
4. What will the results show? When will I know? (1, 2)

Similar to the patient concerns about illness, physicians can assume that each patient wants to know the answers to these additional unspoken questions. Direct, simple language and honesty are helpful approaches in answering these questions. If a test is going to hurt, it is important to let the patient know in advance. Terms like "discomfort" and "pressure" should not be used for experiences that most

CLINICAL VIGNETTE 6.3

"Ms. Robinson, the test we need to do next to understand what's causing your blood problems is called a bone marrow biopsy, which I want to schedule for this Friday. It's the only way we can find out why your bone marrow is not producing healthy cells. I will biopsy, or take a sample, of marrow from your back hipbone with a strong needle. Because the needle needs to go through bone, it is painful. I use some local anesthetic—like the novocaine you get for dental work—but it will still hurt, and you may want to have some pain medicine before and after the procedure. (We'll review your pain medicine prescription in a minute.) You may also want to have your husband there with you to hold your hand and give you emotional support. The whole procedure takes about 20 minutes, and though you will be pretty sore, you will still be able to walk and drive the next day. The samples from the needle go to the lab, and we get information back after two working days. I want you to call me next Tuesday after noon, and I will have that lab report then. There may be a chance we'd want to send the sample out to a specialty lab, but we'll discuss that when we talk on Tuesday."

To a pediatric patient: "Jimmy, I want to swab—wipe with this big cotton swab—way back in your mouth to see if you have strep throat like your sister. This way we'll know if you need medicine or not. The swab feels funny and some kids say it hurts or makes them gag, but I will be really quick—and when it's over, it's over. OK?"

people would consider genuinely painful (see Vignette 6.3). Understandably, the patient–physician relationship suffers when patients feel that a physician has misrepresented the test or treatment, or that they were "tricked" into a painful experience. The patient also needs to know about

CLINICAL VIGNETTE 6.4

Mrs. Gottschalk, is there anything else about the diagnosis and treatment of nasal polyps that you would like to ask me about?
Mr. Milos, we've talked about a lot of different things about your glaucoma. What do you think is most important?
Because the change in medicine that we talked about is pretty complicated, I'd like for you to repeat to me what we planned so that I can be sure I was clear.

the "downsides" of a procedure or treatment to give informed consent; this is an ethical and legal requirement.

After addressing the patients' unspoken questions and offering them the information they need, physicians can supplement a patient's education by checking to see whether he or she has other questions and whether the patient has a good understanding of the information (2) (see Vignette 6.4).

Patients who have their questions answered and even anticipated are more likely to understand and adhere to the physician's recommendations. With less anxiety and more confidence that their physician truly understands their situation (including their unspoken fears and questions), patients are also more likely to be satisfied and to have better medical outcomes.

KEY POINTS

1. Patient education can dramatically improve adherence and outcomes.
2. Patients generally want to know many things about their illness but are unable or reluctant to ask directly.
3. Physicians can anticipate many of the questions patients will have about their illnesses and about medical interventions.

4. Patient questions are best answered as honestly, directly, and simply as possible.

REFERENCES

1. Keller VF, Carroll JG. A new model for physician–patient communication. Patient Educ Couns 1994;23:134–140.
2. Bayer Institute for Health Care Communication. Clinician–patient communication to enhance health outcomes: a workshop manual. New Haven, CT: Bayer Institute, 1998.
3. Stewart MA Effective physician-patient communication and health outcomes: a review. Can Med Assoc J 1995;152:1423–1433.
4. Buckalew LW, Salis RE. Patient compliance and medication prescription. J Clin Psychol 1986;41:49–53.
5. How to improve patient safety: "Ahh" shouldn't be the only thing you say at the doctor's office. Chicago: National Patient Safety Foundation, 2001.
6. Waitzen H. Doctor-patient communication: implications of social science research. JAMA 1984;252:2441–2446.
7. Miyaji NT. The power of compassion: truth telling among American doctors in the care of dying patients. Soc Sci Med 1993;36:249–264.
8. Kravitz RL, Hays RD, Donald Sherbourne C, et al. Recalls of recommendations and adherence to advice among patients with chronic medical conditions. Arch Intern Med 1993;153: 1869–1878.
9. Hadlow J, Pitts M. The understanding of common health terms by doctors, nurses and patients. Soc Sci Med 1991;32: 193–196.

7

Enlist

"Enlistment" is the fourth "E" of the four effective communication techniques. Enlistment means collaboration—the sharing of decision making—and is critical for patient adherence (1, 2).

Many patients and physicians are used to the physician making all the decisions. Although this seems to make sense from the point of view of medical training, typical patient adherence to medical treatment is so low that something more than medical expertise needs to occur in the physician–patient encounter (3). By educating patients (as discussed in Chapter 6) and then involving them in the decision making, physicians can improve patient satisfaction and adherence, and, therefore, medical outcomes.

The first part of enlisting a patient in his or her medical care is an invitation. Some patients are used to being "passive," expecting the physician to take charge because of past experiences with "paternalistic" physicians. A first step in enlisting a patient is also a part of the education process—asking the patient what he or she believes is the problem and the treatment. By eliciting the patient's perception of the underlying problem and opinion about the efficacy of treatment, the physician can understand where the potential adherence roadblocks lie. If a patient has a self-diagnosis that differs dramatically from the physician's assessment, adherence is unlikely without collaboration and compromise (1, 2) (see Vignette 7.1).

CLINICAL VIGNETTE 7.1

Patient: Doc, I think this cough is just allergies and old age. Everyone in my family sounded like this when they reached 50. I just need a few days off and maybe an allergy inhaler.
MD: Allergies could certainly play a role here. I think your smoking could also contribute, and there's also a chance there is an infection in your lungs that is causing mischief as well.
Patient: Well, I don't want to take any antibiotics—they make me sick.
MD: I have a number of ideas for treatment that could be helpful. Let's look at the different options together.

There are other practical enlistment techniques. The first is to simplify the prescription whenever possible (1, 2). Patient adherence to medications decreases dramatically when they are asked to take more than one daily dose. Patients who have complicated problems—such as high blood pressure, obesity, smoking, and borderline diabetes—often need multiple recommendations for diet, exercise, medication, and behavior changes. Such patients cannot retain and adhere to a "laundry list" of physician recommendations. A more effective approach is to ask patients, based on what they know to be the problems, what single thing they would be willing to work on in the interval between visits, and then collaborate on some realistic and specific goals for that period (see Vignette 7.2).

Other approaches a physician can use include adapting a treatment regimen to a patient's lifestyle and getting the patient's feedback on the feasibility of a treatment program. Many patients have work and family schedules that interfere with regular meals or routine medication times. Another effective enlistment technique is to write out the directions or instructions, as most patients retain less than

CLINICAL VIGNETTE 7.2

MD: Mr. Beardsly, we've reviewed some of your health concerns and my ideas about ways to improve your breathing. Of the different things we've talked about, which seems most "doable" to you right now?
Patient: Doctor, I don't think I can do anything about my weight or about my job and the smoke I have to deal with there. I've tried before and I think I'm stuck there for now.
MD: OK, is there anything else that you think you *could* try?
Patient: Well, I could try and use the breathing inhaler more like you want me to. I've sort of neglected that—leaving it in the car at night and not really inhaling when I do use it.
MD: I think that's a good thing to try. Can you try to use the breathing inhaler three times a day, about the same time each day?
Patient: Yeah, except I don't always get a break at work and I'm embarrassed to use it in front of other people. I can put my wife in charge of the times I'm at home. She's a real stickler for these sorts of things and would probably enjoy being in charge.

50% of what they heard during an average visit. Handouts personalized with highlighters and margin notes are also very useful (1, 2).

Obviously, some treatment interventions are not negotiable. These include anything that puts the patient or others at undue risk or compromises the physician's professional integrity. Examples include prescribing medications that are not medically needed or agreeing with a seriously ill patient to discontinue a potentially beneficial treatment (see Vignette 7.3).

CLINICAL VIGNETTE 7.3

Ms. Su, I am not comfortable prescribing narcotics for your condition, and I have to decline.

Mr. Charles, I understand that you and your wife don't agree with the pneumonia diagnosis I gave you and that you wish to discontinue the antibiotics. I cannot agree to do this with you, because I feel you would be at a very high risk for a worsening of the infection. Some people even die of untreated pneumonia. Because you are competent to make medical decisions for yourself, no one could force you into taking treatment you don't want to have. This can be your choice, but I cannot agree. I'd like for you to get a second opinion, and to see if there is anything else you would like to know about treatments and alternatives.

There are often additional barriers to adherence unique to each patient. Physicians can prepare for these with patients and further improve understanding and adherence. These barriers can be addressed after they are elicited from patients (1, 2) (see Vignette 7.4).

Other predictable barriers to patient adherence are side effects, missed doses, and patient lack of motivation. For each of these, a physician can educate a patient on what to expect and how best to prepare. The problems won't go away, but a prepared patient is more likely to effectively manage the setbacks and continue to adhere to the prescribed treatment (1, 2).

CLOSING

At the end of each visit, the physician needs to close the interview. Some patients need advance notice that the visit is wrapping up in the next few minutes. Some medical

CLINICAL VIGNETTE 7.4

MD: What might get in the way of your physical therapy program?
Patient: Work gets sort of squirrelly some days, and I have to put in overtime and then I can't get to the gym.
MD: What are some ways around that?
Patient: I guess I could talk to my boss about "Doctor's Orders" and make sure I get regular hours.
MD: Anything else?
Patient: I could ask my husband to babysit during nap-time on a weekend day and go on a Saturday afternoon if I miss a regular day.
MD: Sounds good. When we next meet, let's see how those two ideas have worked to get you to PT four times a week.

offices inadvertently allow the medical doctor to "disappear," and leave it to a nurse to announce the end of the appointment. This can be disconcerting, even alienating, for patients. Spending a few moments to close the interview allows both the physician and the patient to summarize the diagnosis and treatment plans. The physician also may identify the next step in the treatment plan, which could be a laboratory test, a phone call, or a follow-up visit to check the effects of a new medication. Closing also provides a clear ending to the interpersonal exchange that just occurred. Many physicians cement the positive rapport from a visit with a handshake and some friendly words (2) (see Box 7.1).

BOX 7.1

It's been nice seeing you. Thanks for coming in today.

I hope you feel better soon. Take good care of yourself and that beautiful baby!

Since I won't be seeing you for a few months, I'll wish you a happy holiday season now.

CLINICAL VIGNETTE 7.5

Those are some good questions on your list—I wish we had more time today so we could go over them. I'd like for you to ask Mary at the reception desk to make a photocopy of the list so I can have it in your chart for our next appointment.

I can see you are feeling upset right now. Let's take a few moments to find out where those tears are coming from and then perhaps we can identify what might be helpful.

Sometimes problems occur at the end of a patient's appointment. The patient may, just at that moment, remember a list of questions in his or her pocket or may burst into tears. There is of course no single right way to manage "end of interview surprises." When in doubt, the physician may need to spend a few extra minutes assessing the problem at hand and deferring outstanding issues to another, more appropriate, time (see Vignette 7.5).

KEY POINTS

1. When patients actively participate in medical decision making, adherence improves.
2. Practical enlistment techniques include simplifying the regimen, tailoring the treatment to the patient and identifying potential obstacles.
3. Closing the interview allows for summary, clarification, and cementing of the positive rapport.

REFERENCES

1. Keller VF, Carroll JG. A new model for physician–patient communication. Patient Educ Couns 1994;23:134–140.

2. Bayer Institute for Health Care Communication. Clinician–patient communication to enhance health outcomes: a workshop manual. West Haven, CT: Bayer Institute, 1998.
3. DiMatteo MR, Reiter RC, Gambone JC. Enhancing medication adherence through communication and informed collaborative choice. Health Commun 1994;6:253–265.

8

Getting Feedback

Although books and manuals on communication skills can be helpful to a student or physician interested in learning the most effective patient interview, true skill building happens in real-life encounters. This is why most U.S. medical schools include in vivo demonstrations and practice of interview skills with patients as part of a student's education in clinical skills (1). In educational research, feedback has been found to be the *most* effective way to improve achievement (2). Because of its value in achieving effective communication skills, feedback is widely used in the training of all health care professionals (3).

MODELING

> People seldom improve when they have no other model than themselves to copy after.—Gold Smith

There are two primary ways someone learns a new skill: 1) by observing others or 2) by practicing and getting feedback. Observation of communication skills in a master clinician is a rich and valuable experience. The observer is able to consider new ways of approaching patients and patient problems. Some physicians have a difficult time at first expressing friendliness and empathy to patients. Observing a warm, caring interaction is an effective way to learn how to appropriately express empathy. Sometimes the warmest and most heartfelt expressions of kindness and caring can be observed as nonverbal communication—a touch or an understanding nod. At times, physicians will find themselves learning a new approach in empathy or engagement from a nurse or medical student.

Not every physician–patient encounter demonstrates effective skills. Some physicians have poor skills, and unfortunately they model these skills to students and residents. The careful observer, however, will notice the negative effects on the relationship with the patient and the patient's medical treatment, and will deduce from this what does *not* work. For example, patients will close up after multiple early interruptions or decreases in eye contact, and they will not participate in the interview when the interviewer is detached or unempathic. The goal, however, is that students and physicians interested in developing effective skills will identify good models, and have the opportunity to observe effective patient interviews and discuss them with the interviewer later.

COACHING

The most important feedback any interviewer will ever get is from a colleague or supervisor who can give specific information in a supportive, informative manner. Because this approach does not usually include a formal evaluation, it can be considered "coaching" (4). Coaching can apply to any part of interviewing performance—actual patient interactions, role play, or standardized patient interviews.

Effective coaching occurs when a learner gets feedback in a supportive setting, and when the feedback is so specific that he or she can truly use it to improve skills. We will discuss the five key elements to effective coaching and feedback, and look at a transcript of a coaching session.

Key Elements to Effective Feedback

1. *Agree on the format.* For example, coaching could focus on reviews of videotape or observed patient interviews. Feedback sessions can occur as closed-door individual meetings or group sessions with other learners.
2. *Agree on goals.* Learners may wish to focus on certain skills during different parts of their training. Specific goals are most helpful in the feedback process. Examples of specific communication goals are "I will not interrupt the patient in the first 60 seconds of the interview" or "I will convey warmth and caring in greeting the patient."
3. *Start with self-assessment.* Each feedback session on a specific performance should start with the learner first assessing his or her performance. This self-assessment relates to the stated goals as well as to any other relevant observations about performance.
4. *Structure the feedback.* Each feedback session should include a structure, by breaking it up into four parts (4):
   A. These are the things you do well and should continue to do . . .
   B. These are some things you need to do more of to improve your effectiveness . . .
   C. These are some things you need to do less of to improve your effectiveness . . .
   D. These are some things you need to consider changing to improve your effectiveness . . .
5. Be as specific and concrete as possible in each part of the assessment.

"Constructive" Feedback

It is human nature to avoid directly giving and getting negative feedback, which is one of the reasons the euphemism "constructive" feedback is often used. The confrontational aspect of giving less than glowing feedback to students and subordinates has led to the use of "impersonal" forms that avoid confrontation or grade inflation (5). Without information on weaknesses, however, the potential for improvement is seriously stunted. Most students, when asked, desire to have *all* the feedback they can obtain on their performance.

Structuring four-part feedback into the format described above allows for more freedom in communicating all aspects of performance by specifically addressing areas of good and poor performance. One of the advantages of this format is that it is simple and clear for both the coach and the learner. Another major advantage is that this format first emphasizes positive feedback, the things that the learner does well. This allows the coach and the learner to build a feeling of shared purpose (see Vignette 8.1).

Although the process is not exactly comfortable at first, over time a coach and learner can scrutinize interview behaviors (including grooming, language, and skills) productively because it is in the context of a nonjudgmental and helpful relationship. Many students and physicians consider negative feedback much more valuable than positive feedback because they believe (and are probably right) that they already know what they are good at.

Finding and "Making" a Coach

Coaches are often supervisors—faculty, senior colleagues, or department leaders who are used to evaluating junior colleagues. However, the "rank" of the coach is not as important as his or her willingness to take on the role. The best coach is the person who shares the learner's goals of excellent interviewing skills (and who may already have such skills). This type of coach also is willing to commit to the time needed to observe the entire patient interaction (not just a fragment of an interview), and then systematically offer you observations and feedback. Sometimes the best coaches are peers, because peers can relate to the challenges of everyday practice and the need to improve

as you came into the room, you were so focused on your patient that you walked right past the sink.
Learner: Whoops. I almost never forget that.
Coach: Right. Another thing I thought could be increased was eye contact. After the first handshake, I thought I saw you "retreat" a little. The way you rolled around on the stool made it hard for him to really catch your eye.
Learner: You know, you're right about that. I like to ride around on those stools because I get restless, but I never thought about eye contact with that.
Coach: I think it could be a little hard, if your patients are sitting on the exam table, to keep you in sight, so to speak. Another thing I thought you could increase during the interview was some patient education. This patient is on a fairly complex treatment plan, and I don't know if *I* could keep track of the meds he has to take. Of course, you may have already given him lots of information in the past and I just didn't get to observe that in this interview.
Learner: I think we did a pretty good job of that a few months ago.
Coach: And his meds are the same?
Learner: Pretty much.
Coach: Good. OK, let's move on to *things to consider doing less of to increase your effectiveness.* I agree with your comments about the chart getting in the way. I wonder if you "parked" the rolling stool or switched to a stationary chair, whether you could use the corner of the counter there to put the chart on and keep it out of the line between you and the patient.
Learner: I could try that. It might be hard to take notes since I'm left-handed.
Coach: Oh. Impossible to take notes if you're left-handed. How about using a supplies cabinet, moved around to your left side, to put the chart on for notes?

Learner: That would work better than the c[illegible] These offices weren't built for lefties.

Coach: That was all I had noted for things to do les[illegible] of. Now the last part is *things to consider doing differently.* One thing I noticed was that you didn't have a pen and had to stop the interview and leave the room to ask the nurse for one. I'd just recommend having a couple in your pocket, or stocking the drawers in the exam room. I also noticed the last part of the interview, when you started to sign off, he had that deep sigh and hung his head. What could have happened differently at that point?

Learner: I could have stopped walking out of the door.

Coach: What else?

Learner: I guess I could have asked if something was wrong.

Coach: How could you have done that?

Learner: I have no idea.

Coach: What about something like this: "Mr. Phillips, I'm wondering if something is bothering you right now?"

Learner: And if he denies it?

Coach: You can gently confront him with your observations: "When I see you sigh and look down like that, I think you must be feeling bad about something—please tell me what it is."

Learner: And then what?

Coach: He may tell you what's on his mind, and you may need to respond immediately. Or maybe you can reassure him and plan to talk about it more later. He may not tell you what's on his mind, but he'll know that you were listening and seeing he was upset.

Learner: Maybe next time I can bring it up.

Coach: That a great idea. Any questions about the feedback we reviewed just now?

Learner: No, I think I see your points. I've got some new things to try.

skills. Some coaches are standardized patients; others are hired consultants who are available to physicians who are highly motivated to improve their patient satisfaction and outcome. Large medical centers sometimes have education departments that provide coaching to staff clinicians.

Finding a suitable and available coach is only part of the task. Most supervisors are unfamiliar with a nonevaluative approach to feedback. Potential coaches need to find out what a learner is hoping for and whether they can provide it with their available time and skills. Learners can best prepare a potential coach by reviewing with him or her the material on coaching from this chapter and preparing a four-page or four-part feedback tool following the proposed structure above to be used in feedback sessions. They can also be specific about what time commitment they would like to have from the potential coach.

Significant effort and time are required to develop coaching for feedback. Because feedback is the most effective way to improve achievement, motivated students and physicians will find their efforts well invested.

VIDEOTAPED FEEDBACK

Videotaping interviews is an important means to observe oneself and to get detailed feedback from coaches. Most people are uncomfortable having a videotape recorder pointed at them, and dislike watching themselves on a television monitor. It is very natural to resist opportunities to videotape patient encounters, but there is no adequate substitute for such real-life feedback. With a videotaped interview a student can see firsthand how he or she looks to others. Many people are surprised by small, possibly distracting habits they may see revealed for the first time on tape—for example, dramatic hand gestures, pained facial expressions, or chewing on a pen.

In a study that used video feedback to teach a different type of skill, laryngoscopy, medical students were asked to report their performance before and after watching their performance on videotape. The feedback they received from watching themselves on videotape changed their impressions. Only one student felt that his technique was suboptimal prior to watching the video playback, whereas 10 of the 26 (38%) students felt this was true after watching the tape of their performance. Students also tended to underestimate the amount of time they had spent on the procedure compared to the actual time they were able to measure on the playback. Although 27% of the students felt the taping was a distraction, they all felt it was a useful educational experience (6). A taped patient interview is more complex than a single procedure, but it gives observers abundant information on their communication techniques as well as on their general appearance and demeanor.

The keys to making and viewing a useful videotape for feedback include:

1. Getting the patient's signed consent.
2. Having adequate audio (although even muted tapes give quite a bit of information to the observer).
3. Using a stopwatch to time different parts of the interview when viewing the tape (such as the time interval before the patient is first interrupted).
4. Agreeing on a feedback procedure in advance if working with a coach.
5. Reviewing the tape in a private, noncritical environment (7).

Many students and physicians keep a library of tapes of their interviews to review their progress over time and refresh their memories of particular "traps" or old habits they might lapse into. Audiotaped interviews are another option, but they lack the nonverbal interactions and thus many of the benefits of the videotape.

STANDARDIZED PATIENTS

Some schools offer students the opportunity to work with standardized patients. These "patients" are trained actors who portray an illness and then give feedback from the perspective of the patient. Standardized patient programs may use hidden video equipment that allows for the taping of interviews and for a review with the "patient" afterward. This type of feedback has been highly rated by students (3). Standardized patients may also evaluate student performance with feedback forms.

The use of standardized patients is becoming very popular in medical education and is a valuable opportunity for any student enrolled in a school or a program that allows for practice of interviewing (and physical examination) skills. Data on student communication skill development show that feedback from standardized patients was at least as effective as faculty feedback in improving students' skills (8).

Standardized patients are also popular for clinical evaluation exercises among medical schools, residencies, and national board examinations. Some students do not get opportunities to practice with the format of a standardized patient and are at a relative disadvantage in these examinations. One way to offset this is the use of role play. This is usually done by having a colleague or supervisor play the role of a patient in an interview; feedback is provided from the perspective of the "patient" and from videotape. Role play is most effective when the person playing the role of the patient has an actual individual in mind, and speaks and feels in the place of that individual.

When there are few opportunities to enlist anyone in role play, feedback from actual patients can be particularly valuable.

PATIENT FEEDBACK

Another mechanism for obtaining feedback on skills in the "real world" is by asking the patient. Many students and physicians are uncomfortable asking for "criticism" from their patients. A physician could also ask, if a patient looks upset (or relieved), "I wonder if there is something I just said or didn't say that made you feel upset (or better)."

CLINICAL VIGNETTE 8.2

At the opening of the interview (following the greeting):

"Today's visit is perhaps going to be a bit different. I'm asking my patients for feedback on some of my communication skills. If you can bear this in mind while we talk today, I'll check back and see if there are specific things I say or do that either are helpful to you or that you think I could change."

At the end of the interview (following the closing of patient-related topics):

"We are at the end of today's time, and I'd like to take a few moments and see what feedback you have for me. What are some of the things you think I do well—things that worked for you—with my communication style?"

"Now what are a few things you think I could do differently—things that would have helped you in some way during this last appointment?"

Answers to these types of questions can provide information both about the interviewer and the patient. A physician may *also ask for more general feedback* (see Vignette 8.2).

There are a variety of questionnaires used in research and clinical practice that measure patient satisfaction and a patient's assessment of the rapport or the therapeutic alliance. Some physicians design their own questionnaires to target specific information about themselves and their practice. The feedback from most questionnaires gives information to physicians about what they do well. Patients are also usually willing to describe some things they did not like about their doctor's visit, thus giving physicians information about what they need to improve. Although questionnaires don't allow for the opportunity to follow up with more questions (or apologize for an unintended lapse), they can be given to a patient by someone other than the physician and filled out confidentially at the patient's leisure. Some patients may be reluctant to tell their physician directly about a communication problem from the visit, but are willing to write it down on an "impersonal" piece of paper after they have said goodbye to the doctor. A patient questionnaire designed by Steine and colleagues (9) asks the patient to rate the following: quality of the connection with the physician, use of time during the interview, experiences with non-physician staff, and the patient's emotions immediately after each visit. This and other questionnaires can be adapted to a specific clinician's setting and to specific concerns (10, 11).

KEY POINTS

1. Feedback is the most important factor in changing performance.
2. Exemplary clinicians can model behaviors that cannot be learned from books or lectures.
3. Coaching with a structured feedback format is a useful way of obtaining both positive and negative information about one's performance.
4. Other sources of feedback are videotaping, standardized patients, and questionnaires.

REFERENCES

1. Novack DH, Volk G, Drossman DA, Lipkin M Jr. Medical interviewing and interpersonal skills teaching in US medical schools. Progress, problems, and promise. JAMA 1993;269: 2101–2105.
2. Hattie JA. Measuring the effects of schooling. Aust J Educ 1990;36:5–13.
3. Sachdeva AK. Use of effective feedback to facilitate adult learning. J Cancer Educ 1996;11:106–118.
4. Bayer Institute for Health Care Communications. CPC faculty leader's manual. West Haven, CT: Bayer Institute, 1997.

5. Coletti LM. Difficulty with negative feedback: face-to-face evaluation of junior medical student clinical performance results in grade inflation. J Surg Res 2000;90:82–87.
6. Kardash K, Tessler MJ. Videotape feedback in teaching laryngoscopy. Can J Anaesth 1997;44:54–58.
7. Lui P, Miller E, Herr G, et al. Videotape reliability: a method for evaluation of a clinical performance examination. J Med Educ 1980;55:713–715.
8. Vannatta JB, Smith KR, Crandall S, et al. Comparison of standardized patients and faculty in teaching medical interviewing. Acad Med 1996;71:1360–1362.
9. Steine S, Finset A, Laerum E. A new, brief questionnaire (PEQ) developed in primary care for measuring patients' experience of interaction, emotion and consultation outcome. Fam Pract 2001;18:410–418.
10. Luborsky L, Barber JP, Siqueland L, et al. The Revised Helping Alliance Questionnaire (HAQ-II): psychometric properties. J Psychother Pract Res 1996;5:260–271.
11. Flocke SA. Measuring attributes of primary care: development of a new instrument. J Fam Prac 1997;45:64–74.

9

Special Situations

In the practice of medicine, all physicians are faced with "special situations," especially early in their careers. Over time, most physicians learn strategies that allow them to manage 99% of their patients with confidence. Some specialties have a focus on special situations, such as managing "bad news" among oncologists. This chapter offers some tools and suggestions for developing effective ways to communicate with patients who are in special circumstances or who require specific types of communication skills.

WORKING WITH LANGUAGE AND CULTURAL BARRIERS

Most physicians enjoy variety in their patient population. Different age groups and patient personalities can add to the richness of a day practicing medicine. At times, patient diversity becomes a challenge, as when patients do not share a common language with the physician or have very different cultural beliefs that impact on their medical care.

Language barriers can be partial, where some words and phrases are known; or barriers can be complete, where there is no shared language. It is human nature to smile and nod when someone is trying to communicate with you, despite a language barrier. Smiling and nodding, of course, do not mean that someone understands—just that he or she wishes to show respect and is eager to please.

Due to the false impression of understanding, partial language barriers can be more difficult than complete ones. In these circumstances, the physician has two options: use an interpreter to confirm understanding or double-check *every few sentences* for comprehension. Both options are time consuming, and at times an interpreter may not be available.

When interpreters are available, they are invaluable. The best interpreters are unrelated to the patient (and therefore unlikely to inhibit the disclosure of sensitive information) and share a similar cultural background. Effective patient communication with an interpreter includes greeting the patient in his or her own language, if possible, and making eye contact with the patient and not with the interpreter when asking questions. Some interpreters can give not only verbatim translations but also can give a cultural context for how usual or unusual the patient's problems are. For example, a patient may feel ill after eating a certain food on a certain day. The interpreter can report the symptoms, and can also describe a taboo or religious prohibition against that food that may contribute to the patient's symptoms.

Even when they are fluent in the culture and language of a patient, interpreters have limitations. Some languages lack vocabulary for certain medical terms. The Hmong language, for example, lacks a word for "gallbladder," and interpreters of this language have to be creative to translate terms such as "endoscopy" or "CT-guided biopsy." Before the patient can receive education about his or her illness and treatment plan, physicians must first educate the interpreters about it and ensure their understanding.

More subtle, and possibly more threatening, to good patient care are cultural barriers. Different cultures and subcultures carry beliefs and traditions about illness and medicine that can significantly impact the patient's understanding and adherence to treatment. Unless a physician specifically asks about these beliefs and traditions, patients are unlikely to disclose the reasons they did not understand

BOX 9.1

What do you call the problem?

What do you think caused the problem?

Why do you think it started when it did?

How does the sickness work?

How severe is the sickness? What is its course?

What kind of treatment should it receive? What results will come from this treatment?

What are the chief problems from this sickness?

What do you fear most about this sickness? (1)

---

or follow a treatment plan. Box 9.1 shows the gold standard of questions described by Kleinman to help uncover a patient's cultural model; they are invaluable in promoting understanding and adherence in medical treatment involving people of different cultures.

The same questions that are used when cultural differences threaten to block effective communication and understanding can also be helpful when no obvious cultural difference appears yet a patient and a physician seem to be at an impasse in agreeing on a treatment plan or when a patient has demonstrated very poor adherence to previously prescribed plan.

A richer understanding of the impact of language and cultural barriers on patient care can be gained through reading. The book *The Spirit Catches You and You Fall Down* chronicles the life story of an immigrant child and the problems both the patient and the physicians experienced because of cultural differences (2).

GIVING BAD NEWS

No physician wants to give bad news to patients, but most accept it as part of their duty. There are special skills that can help effectively communicate bad news. In addition, the nonspecific qualities of engaging and empathizing with the patient are crucial in delivering such information.

A six-step protocol for giving bad news has been widely used in teaching clinicians communication skills (3). The protocol has a mnemonic: "SPIKES" (4).

1. *Establish the **S**etting.* The impact of bad news can be improved when the patient feels comfortable with the setting. An appropriate setting is one in which the physician has allotted sufficient time and will not feel or look rushed, when a significant other can be present (if desired), and when the patient is not distracted by pain or interruptions.
2. *Solicit the patient's **P**erception of the problem.*
3. ***I**nvite the patient to control the information flow.* Open with "I have the results of the tests [surgery, etc.]" and then allow the patient to formulate questions.
4. *Provide **K**nowledge to the patient.* Give information in digestible pieces, with as much clarity and truthfulness as possible.
5. ***E**mpathize with expressed emotions.* Also inquire about unexpressed emotions: "This clearly isn't the news we were hoping for. How are you emotionally?"
6. ***S**ummarize* the information discussed.

A key principle to giving bad news is to be truthful. Historically, physicians have at times protected their patients from the truth. It is no longer acceptable, legally or ethically, to withhold information relevant to a patient's diagnosis or prognosis (5).

Giving bad news is an opportunity for most physicians to be especially aware of nonverbal communication. Eye contact, facial expression, and appropriate touching—such as on the hand or the arm—can show without words how much the physician cares and how sad he or she feels about the diagnosis. The experience of seeing and feeling the physician's empathy can dramatically change the patient's experience of bad news.

Dying patients present personal and professional challenges to most physicians. Medical school rarely prepares anyone for the experience of caring for a dying person. In fact, medical culture often frames death as a treatment failure. As a result, physicians are led to retreat from their feelings of sadness (and sometimes shame) into objective "science." Although this may temporarily protect the physician, it does not meet the patient's needs. In fact, the patient–physician relationship may benefit from a visible emotional response in the physician. It informs patients that the physician is sharing in their experience as another human being and can make the dying experience less lonely. The process of identifying with the patient's suffering and loss is also an important part of a physician's ability to come to terms over time with his or her role in a patient's death (6).

PSYCHIATRIC PATIENTS

When medical students pick nonpsychiatric residencies, they may think that they have selected a practice of medicine that does not include psychiatric patients. After a short period of practice, however, most physicians realize that psychiatric patients are present in all medical settings. In primary care, up to one-fourth of all patients have symptoms that meet criteria for a psychiatric diagnosis, and another 15% have some symptoms but do not meet diagnostic criteria (7). Typical psychiatric problems in the general medical population are depression, anxiety, somatoform disorders, and substance abuse.

Despite the high prevalence of these disorders, many patients are not diagnosed because they report physical, not psychiatric complaints. Often, patients with undiagnosed psychiatric disorders are found to be "difficult" patients who do not respond well to treatment or who have higher than usual health care use, needing more frequent appointments and more overall treatment (8).

All of the basic communication skills described in earlier chapters are useful when a patient reports with psychiatric complaints. When soliciting a patient's understanding or

CLINICAL VIGNETTE 9.1

MD: Ms. Abbot, what do you think your sleep and energy problems are from?
Patient: I don't know. My concentration is bad too, and I'm really crabby all the time.
MD: Sometimes those problems happen with depression. Do you think you might be depressed?
Patient: I don't know. I just know I'm really struggling.
MD: I suspect depression is at least a part of this, and I'd like to offer you some information about depression and how we treat it. It's a very treatable illness, and many people get relief from counseling, medication, or both. Have you ever had a diagnosis for depression in the past?
Patient: No, but my mother had it. She took some pills that seemed to help.
MD: Let's start with discussing medication treatments, OK?

explanation of the problem, the physician may need to gently suggest that the underlying symptoms represent a psychiatric disorder (see Vignette 9.1). Most people are reluctant to offer psychiatric reasons for their symptoms because of personal and cultural stigma surrounding mental disorders.

The most important aspect of communication with patients about psychiatric problems is to identify the problems. The majority of patients who kill themselves have seen a primary care doctor in the hours or weeks before the suicide. Rarely did the physician detect an underlying psychiatric problem (9, 10). To increase their detection of psychiatric problems and diagnoses, physicians can benefit from continuing medical education, consultation, and screening tools.

Most specialties have annual state and national meetings that provide opportunities to learn or refresh areas

CLINICAL VIGNETTE 9.2

MD: Ms. Johnson, from what you've told me, it seems like you have been deeply depressed for a while now. Have you ever felt so sad or hopeless that you have had thoughts of death or dying?
Patient: From time to time . . .
MD: Are you having any thoughts like that today?
Patient: Well, maybe not so much today.
MD: Have you had any plans on how you might hurt yourself?
Patient: I sort of thought about the cellar. There's a rope there and a beam.
MD: Hmm. It sounds like your thoughts have gone to planning. I'd like to see about getting you some extra help, because I'm worried about your depression. I want to make some phone calls and need to step out. Will you be comfortable waiting here for a few more minutes? Thanks.

of knowledge and skills. To stay fresh in the diagnosis and treatment of common psychiatric problems, most physicians can choose an educational activity each year in this area. In addition, many physicians benefit from relationships with colleagues in their community who are practicing other specialties. Every non-psychiatrist should have a relationship with a colleague in psychiatry who can provide both informal (over the phone) and formal (patient referral) consultations.

In addition to training and consultation, there are screening instruments available. These are usually questionnaires a patient fills out in the waiting room before a scheduled appointment. Some screens are for depression, such as the Beck Depression Inventory (11) or Patient Health Questionnaire-9 (12). Others screen more generally for psychiatric symptoms and problems in living, such as the

CLINICAL VIGNETTE 9.3

MD: Well, Mr. Fife, we have almost finished this part of the interview. Now I will ask you some routine questions that I ask everybody. Is there ever a time you hear voices and there is no one there?
Patient: When I get upset or locked up in jail. Sometimes they get really bad.
MD: Tell me more about them.
Patient: Well, they are sometimes really mean and tell me bad things and I don't know what to do.
MD: Do they ever tell you to do things?
Patient: Mostly it's stupid stuff, like to put sugar on my food instead of salt. But sometimes, like last week, they were telling me to hurt somebody bad so I would get hurt. Real screwed up stuff. I hate it.
MD: Is there anything today that you feel they are telling you to do?
Patient: No, they are real quiet today.
MD: It sounds like they can be threatening for you sometimes. I want to tell you about our local mental health clinic, because I think they can help you with this. And I want you to call me if you feel you are losing control.

Primary Care Evaluation of Mental Disorders (PRIME-MD) (13). Patients are usually willing to complete these forms along with the other paperwork required on an annual basis or at their first appointment as a new patient. Nursing and reception staff can score the screening questionnaires and highlight items that the physician needs to notice before seeing a patient, such as the presence of suicidal thoughts. Questionnaires are generally high yield in obtaining important information in a short period of time.

Some patients have severe or acute psychiatric disturbances, such as psychosis or suicidal thoughts and plans (see Vignettes 9.2 and 9.3). Every physician needs to be able to assess the extent of these problems and to know

CLINICAL VIGNETTE 9.4

MD: Mrs. Phillips, that was a lot of information about the test results. How are you doing?
Patient: (gasping) I don't know doctor, I just don't know.
MD: It looks like you are feeling very upset and are having a hard time breathing. [1. Acknowledge.]
MD: Yes.
MD: Let's take a few breaths together. Follow with me. Breathe in 1–2–3–4, and out 1–2–3–4, and in 1–2–3–4, and out 1–2–3–4.
Patient: OK. That's better. I think I can catch my breath again.
MD: When someone feels upset, sometimes it's better to take a break. Would you like to have a few moments to yourself, have a cup of water—or even reschedule for later this week? [2. Give options.]
Patient: No—I'm really OK now. But thanks. Let's go on. I'd like to find out what my test results mean. I'll let you know if I need a break.

where to get emergency help when needed. Handbooks of psychiatry contain additional information on common psychiatric emergencies.

THE "OUT OF CONTROL" PATIENT

Some patients appear to lose emotional control during a medical interview. They may become acutely anxious, tearful, or angry and require careful management by the physician. In general, these acute situations can be managed empathically and effectively with a two-part approach: acknowledge and give options.

Anxious patients may arrive anxious or become anxious during an appointment. Sometimes the anxiety becomes

CLINICAL VIGNETTE 9.5

MD: (after providing information about progression of eye disease) So, how are you doing with all of this?
Patient: (tearful) Fine, I guess.
MD: You look sad to me. [1. Acknowledge.]
Patient: Well, it's terrible. I'm losing my vision and won't be able to drive soon. How would you feel?
MD: I think anyone would feel sad. It's a big loss.
Patient: I was hoping it would get better, not worse.
MD: Of course.
Patient: It's just terrible. (sobs)
MD: Would you like to just sit together for a few moments? Is there something I can bring you? [2. Give options.]
Patient: No. (sobs and blows nose) I'll be OK in a minute.
MD: (sits still, offering eye contact until patient is composed) OK to go on?
Patient: Yeah. Thanks.

a full-blown panic attack, and the patient hyperventilates. Physicians can help a patient in a panic state by leading him or her back to a normal breathing pattern (see Vignette 9.4).

Patients may also become sad and tearful during the course of an interview. Sometimes a physician's job is to simply be there and let the tears flow (see Vignette 9.5). At other times, the assurance that it is perfectly acceptable to feel sad and cry or redirection can be helpful. Tears tend to make physicians anxious and sometimes lead to subtle behaviors (physician hands the patient a box of tissues and turns away) and not-so-subtle behaviors (physician leaves the room and sends in a nurse) that tell the patients that they should not cry. Empathic lapses such as this can damage the patient–physician relationship.

CLINICAL VIGNETTE 9.6

Setting Limits with Angry Patient

MD: I see that you are angry and upset about the prescriptions. [1. Acknowledge.] I understand how it's frustrating, and I think we can work this out. I can work with you here, but I must ask you to lower your voice and stop hitting the walls. [2. Set limit.] Would you like a few minutes to get calm? [3. Give option.]

Patient: (yelling) No! I don't want "a few minutes"! I want my meds!

MD: Let's try to work together. Do you think you can lower your voice?

Patient: You are just screwing around with me! (bangs fist on wall)

MD: I'll step out now. I'll be back in a couple of minutes.

Depending on how well the physician knows the patient, he or she may try to reengage the patient after a few minutes or may bring in some backup to help set limits.

Angry patients present a special challenge because of safety issues. Physicians must always ensure the safety of themselves, the patient, and the staff before proceeding with an interview. The first step in securing safety is setting limits—asking patients to limit their behavior to what is acceptable (see Vignette 9.6). If a patient cannot respond to limit setting and continues threatening or disruptive behavior, such as yelling or banging his or her fist, the physician should stop the interview and obtain backup. A "show of force" of a small group of people (other physicians and support staff) can often help set limits when a patient doesn't respond to a single individual. When a group cannot help set limits and an angry patient's be-havior escalates, security or police may need to be called in.

Patients and families become angry for many different reasons. Sometimes anger is a substitute for fear or sadness, and it dissipates when the underlying emotions are addressed. Some patients have chronic anger problems and need referrals for mental health treatment. Regardless of the source of anger, physicians must put safety first. Following the establishment of safe limits, the physician can acknowledge and give options. For more reading on this topic, Grandinetti (14) offers an in-depth example of an angry patient and provides a "virtual group discussion," which describes possible management approaches.

THE DIFFICULT PHYSICIAN–PATIENT RELATIONSHIP

Every physician practicing medicine will have patients that seem difficult. These are the patients who challenge the physician with nonadherence or inappropriate requests. Sometimes a patient can seem extraordinarily difficult for no clear reason.

There are many signs that a physician is having difficulty with the physician–patient relationship. These include dreading the next appointment (and possibly stretching out the intervals between appointments further than usual), feeling or expressing anger to a patient, or extending special privileges to certain patients (such as giving them a home phone number). Most of the time, the problems in the relationship are treatable.

The best way to improve problematic relationships with patients is to consult with a trusted colleague. Feedback and problem solving might uncover concrete solutions. For example, after hearing a presentation of an "impossible case," a colleague might observe that the patient sounds depressed and might benefit from psychiatric assessment and treatment. Or a colleague might observe that a power struggle appears to be taking place and that improving the patient education and enlistment in treatment planning might improve the relationship. Videotaping a patient

CLINICAL VIGNETTE 9.7

"Mr. Smith, as we have discussed at length, we have had some differences and it seems we should stop working together. I want to be sure that you have good follow up. Here's the number for the other group in town. I will handle anything that comes up for you for the next month. By then you should have been in to see one of my colleagues. Do you have any questions? Let's shake hands. Good luck."

interaction (with patient consent) and enlisting a colleague as a coach (see Chapter 8) could provide clues on how to improve a problematic relationship.

There are times when the physician must ask the patient for his or her thoughts about the relationship: "It seems to me that at times we don't seem to be getting along very well with today's appointment. What do you think we can do differently so we can get along better and work on your problems?" Some patients might be surprised by this frank approach, but they might appreciate the physician's honesty and the message that this is a shared problem and not just the patient's fault. At times, consultation with colleagues and attempts at problem-solving with the patient do not work despite good efforts. Rarely, it is necessary to end a relationship. Any closing of a physician–patient relationship must include referrals to other providers, interim care, documentation in the chart of these provisions, and ideally a handshake with good wishes (see Vignette 9.7).

Some physicians see problematic patient relationships as an opportunity to develop self-awareness. This can happen with individual counseling or with groups, such as Balint groups. Medical educators offer workshops and groups to students and residents, believing that increased self-awareness can improve patient care (15, 16).

Some physician–patient relationships have boundary problems. These types of problems manifest when the role of the physician loses its professionalism. Examples of boundary problems are physicians giving patients special favors, having social contact with patients, or accepting expensive (more than $10) gifts from patients. Often, when a physician behaves in these ways, it is because he or she has become too emotionally involved with the patient. Ultimately, these behaviors degrade the relationship and make the physician less effective as a health care provider. An extreme example of a boundary violation is a sexual relationship with a patient (which is prohibited by medical ethical standards).

Boundary problems for physicians and patients occur when there is poor understanding or acceptance of the limits of the professional relationship. This can occur for either party, but the physician is responsible for maintaining healthy boundaries. When patients challenge boundaries ("Why can't I call you by your first name?"), it is the physician's job to clarify them ("Because this is a professional relationship, I like to go by my professional title"). If physicians sense that they are into a "gray area" of boundaries, they should consult with a colleague or supervisor to confirm the potential lapse and to seek advice on remedying the problem. Sometimes counseling or therapy can help physicians who have a history of boundary problems understand why they have these particular difficulties with patients (17). Rarely are troubled relationships beyond repair, if both parties are motivated to communicate about the boundary difficulties and commit to acceptable "rules."

Challenges in communicating and relationships with patients are as varied as the physicians and patients themselves. With troubled patient relationships, most physicians benefit from consultation with colleagues or other professionals, because others have most likely encountered similar types of problems in their practices. The combination of solid general communication skills and motivation to work out problems can create an extremely effective physician-communicator, in spite of the challenges and obstacles that emerge with patients.

KEY POINTS

1. Cultural and language barriers can be managed by effective use of translators and specific questions to elicit the patient's beliefs about the illness.
2. Bad news is most effectively and empathically communicated with attention to the setting, the patient, and the patient's response.
3. Psychiatric patients may require specific interventions. Management of psychiatric problems depends on identifying underlying diagnoses and problems.
4. Patients who are emotionally out of control can be approached by acknowledgment of the emotion and offering options.
5. Difficult relationships with patients benefit from clarification of roles and expectations. Consultation is an important resource. Some patient relationships require termination.

REFERENCES

1. Kleinman A, Eisenberg L, Good B. Culture, illness and care: clinical lessons from anthropologic and cross-cultural research. Ann Intern Med 1978;88:251–258.
2. Fadiman A. The spirit catches you and you fall down. New York: Farrar, Straus & Giroux, 1997.
3. Baile WF, Kudelka AP, Beale EA, et al. Communication skills training in oncology: description and preliminary outcomes of workshops on breaking bad news and managing patient reactions to illness. Cancer 1999;86:887–897.
4. Buckman R. Breaking bad news: a six-step protocol. In: Buckman R, ed. How to break bad news: a guide for health

care professionals. Baltimore: Johns Hopkins University Press, 1992:65–97.

5. Miyaji N. The power of compassion: truth telling among American doctors in the care of dying patients. Soc Sci Med 1993;36:249–264.
6. Branch WT, Pels RJ, Hafler JP. Medical student's empathic understanding of their patients. Acad Med 1998;73:360–362.
7. Novack DH, Goldberg RJ. Psychiatric problems in primary care patients. J Gen Intern Med 1996;11:56–57.
8. Hahn SR, Kroenke K, Spitzer RL, et al. The difficult patient: prevalence, psychopathology and functional impairment. J Gen Intern Med 1996;11:1–8.
9. Robins E, Gassner S, Kayes J, et al. The communication of suicidal intent: a study of 134 consecutive cases of successful (completed) suicide. Am J Psychiatry 1959;115:724–733.
10. Murphy G. The physician's responsibility for suicide. I. An error of commission. Ann Intern Med 1975;82:301–304.
11. Beck AT, Ward CH, Mendelson M, et al. An inventory for measuring depression. Arch Gen Psychiatry 1961;4:561–571.
12. Kronke K, Spitzer RL, Williams JBW. The PHQ-9: The validity of a brief depression scale. J Gen Intern Med 2001;16:606–613.
13. Spitzer RL, Kroenke K, Williams JB. Validation and utility of a self-report version of PRIME-MD: the PHQ Primary Care Study. JAMA 1999;282:1737–1744.
14. Grandinetti D. Handling patients you wish you didn't have. Med Econ 1997;June 9:142–163.
15. Novack DH, Suchman AL, Clark W, et al. Calibrating the physician: personal awareness and effective patient care. JAMA 1997;278:502–509.
16. Epstein RM. Mindful practice. JAMA 1999;282:833–839.
17. Farber NJ, Novack DH, O'Brien MK. Love, boundaries and the patient–physician relationship. Arch Intern Med 1997;157: 2291–2294.

Index